CHECK ENGINE
LIGHT

TUNING YOUR BODY AND
MIND FOR PERFORMANCE
LONGEVITY

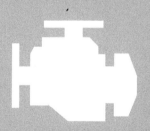

ROB WILSON

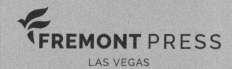
FREMONT PRESS

LAS VEGAS

First published in 2025 by Fremont Press

ISBN-13: 978-1-628605-44-0

Cover and interior design by Kat Lannom

151969226

I dedicate this book to the warfighters. To the many warriors I've had the pleasure and opportunity to work with over the course of my career—you inspired the core of this material. Working with you has been the most humbling and enlightening path I could have asked for.

To all who serve—please keep driving hard. We need you. But don't forget to pull over once in a while and take care of yourselves, too. If you get stuck on the side of the road, you can call on me.

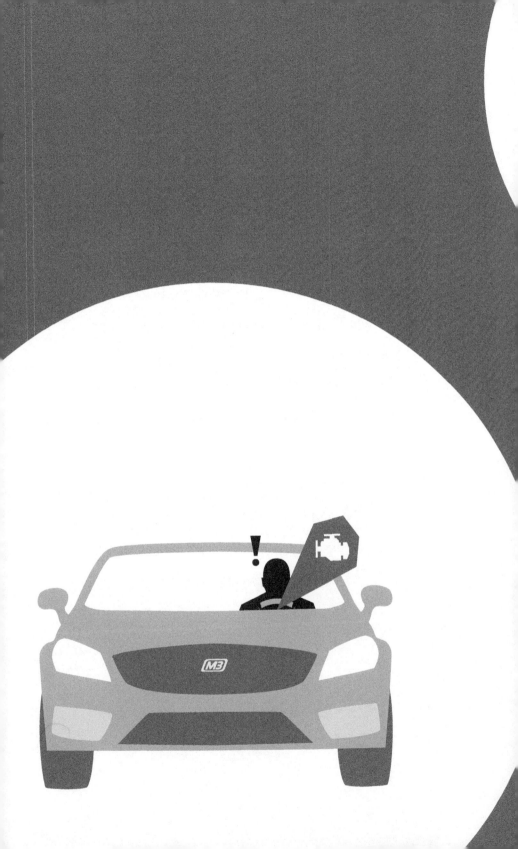

CONTENTS

FOREWORD

Welcome to the age of overwhelm.

Teen athletes are now learning to fuel their bodies from the latest viral TikTok. You can binge three-hour podcasts about human physiology. You can order GLP-1s and HRT during the Super Bowl ad break. You share your HRV, resting heart rate, and body temperature with your group chat before you hop into your red-light bed. Your home is optimized. Your lightbulbs glow red. Your bed is cooled. Your sauna is hot. Your cold plunge is dialed to the latest protocol.

You're still searching for a mitochondrial health supplement that won't interfere with your keto-heavy, time-restricted meal-delivery plan. You've given up alcohol, but you're confused by the algorithm-promoted ads that insist nicotine will help you focus. You're still banana-curious, but worried about what they might do to your A1C.

And your knees still hurt.

You're not thrilled with your body composition. You're more stressed than ever. Your latest DEXA scan shows you're losing muscle and bone mass. And did I mention your knees still hurt—despite those new carbon-plate running shoes?

If you even *kind of* understand the above-coded fitness language, you're holding the right book.

Over the last two decades, human performance has been wildly democratized. We're starting to reckon with the lack of parity in women's sports and address the realities of female physiology. You can grab a decent protein shake at Costco and a surprisingly good protein candy bar at any gas station. You have potential access to the greatest minds in sports, performance, and longevity—right on your phone. You can buy kettlebells and bumper plates at Target.

And yet, most of us still feel like we're missing something.

Because we are.

The promises of the industrial fitness complex aren't leaving our families feeling better. The revolutionary hype of the longevity movement hasn't trickled down to the high school kids in our neighborhoods tearing their ACLs. We're seeing a drop in national obesity rates for the first time in decades—not because we've changed how we eat, play, sleep, or move, but because we've hacked our way to a solution that doesn't actually address the problem.

What we need is a framework. A model. A lens to help us make sense of it all. We need a dashboard—one that can help us better understand our inputs and outputs, our biology and our psychology, our feelings and our potential.

Fortunately, we have Rob Wilson.

This is the part of the foreword where I'm supposed to say I've worked with Rob for over a decade. That he was one of the first coaches I met who intuitively adopted a systems-based approach to working with high performers. That I use the tools he's developed with nearly every athlete, team, and organization I coach.

All of that is true.

Rob is the real deal.

The internet has created an army of self-assured experts, each claiming to live on the bleeding edge of human potential. Social media gives us a daily feed of guru-on-guru violence, clashes of style, and what E. O. Wilson once called "artifacts of scholarship"—impassioned arguments over esoterica that ultimately change nothing, improve nothing, and mean nothing.

Rob stands in stark contrast to all of that.

He's a quiet badass. He works with real people whose complex livelihoods depend on better psycho-physical outcomes. This isn't about aesthetics or biohacking hobbyists obsessing over their HRV data. The gap between what really matters and what has become fitness-as-entertainment is growing wider by the day—and Rob is reaching across the divide with a steady hand.

We're now in the Third Wave of human performance.

If you're a Gen X kid like me, you remember the First Wave—defined by malt-nut PowerBars and first-gen heart rate monitors. Back when we still believed you could outwork the competition. (Spoiler: You can't.)

The Second Wave came crashing in with the rise of YouTube fitness. Suddenly, you didn't need to buy Olympic lifting shoes out of someone's car like it was a drug deal. Training sophistication exploded. So did fitness tribalism, tech fetishism, and—unfortunately—diminishing returns. We leveled up but got lost in the weeds. The question became: *How the hell are we supposed to do all of this?*

The Third Wave is about integration. Simplification. Recalibration. It's the return to context, nuance, and sustainability. It's the long game.

And Rob Wilson is its poster child.

This book is one of the first clear signs that Third Wave thinking is rising out of the chaos. If someone had asked for this book three years ago, it wouldn't have been possible. When Rob called to tell me he was thinking about systematizing his ideas, I nearly begged him to start writing. Then I hung up the phone and quietly thanked the universe that someone else was willing to take this on.

We should treat this book like an indicator species—something that emerges after a catastrophic event to signal that healing is possible. Rob is offering us a way off the shaking mountain.

So consider this your invitation to the next revolution. A chance to reset. A chance to reframe how you understand your body, your mind, and what truly matters.

Let's begin.

—Dr. Kelly Starrett
3x *NYT* Best-Selling Author, Physio, High Performance Coach

PROLOGUE | Lessons from High Performers

High performers have unique programming. In sports, business, and the military, the highest performers are singularly task oriented and forward focused. These rare birds are exceptional at intuiting what information is crucial to the task at hand and disregarding the rest. It's a big part of what completes missions and wins championships. It's what allows high performers to succeed where others fail.

The ability to ignore the periphery and focus on key information coming from the immediate environment is especially important for nullifying physical and emotional discomfort so the job can get done and the goal can be achieved. These folks are typically not emotionally volatile or hypersensitive to pain. In fact, just the opposite: They push pain, frustration, and negativity aside and simply act.

In a fascinating study, researchers compared personality differences among non-athletes, professional athletes, and champions using the Big Five Personality Inventory. The Big Five is a reliable cross-cultural statistical analysis that includes five personality domains: openness, conscientiousness, extraversion, agreeableness, and neuroticism. An easy way to remember them is the acronym OCEAN. The highest predictor of championship performance according to this analysis? Low neuroticism. This trait refers to an individual's tendency to have negative emotions. People who score high in trait neuroticism tend to be more emotionally volatile, are more likely to experience anxiety and depression, and have trouble dealing with stress, especially if it's unexpected. The highest performers showed low neuroticism even when compared to other professionals in the same sport (who already have lower average levels of this trait than the general public). This means the highest performers routinely were the least affected psychologically by negative information from their environment, or, if they were affected, they bounced back rapidly. Being extraordinarily low in the trait neuroticism is what allows the best of the best to hit the mark in stressful, high-stakes situations instead of being ruled by panic and doubt.

It is a superpower for sure, but it's not without its downfalls. Often, lower-threshold issues slip under the radar and don't set off any alarm at all. This is great when it comes to saving lives and winning gold medals but does not alert these individuals to cumulative threats to health and performance longevity. In other words, it's not a single decapitating swipe of the blade that shuts things down, but death by a thousand cuts.

No community better displays the incredible upsides and downsides of being forward focused than the special warfare groups I've had the opportunity to work with over the last few years. No group of people on the planet are tougher or more tenacious. They train and fight through things I might not have believed had I not looked these people in the eyes myself and heard their stories firsthand. They are selected for their ability to endure the most arduous programs the military has to offer. These attributes are further honed to a level of loyalty and grit that is difficult, if not impossible, to find outside of these select groups. Some of my favorite human beings come from this ilk. The character traits of deep loyalty, strength, honor, and fortitude have inspired me in many ways. However, there is often a steep price for them to pay on the other side. Many of these men and women have medical rap sheets a mile long. Career-long habits of going till it's broken and then going some more take an indelible toll on the body and the mind.

This happens to many high performers because of the way they're built. In fact, the Check Engine Light concept that inspired this book, and later became the curriculum I crafted, came about in conversations with retired Navy SEAL Alex Oliver. Alex is the founder of the Continue Mission

Program. In partnership with the Navy SEAL Foundation's Warrior Fitness Program, Continue Mission takes hundreds of active-duty and veteran SEALs through an intensive four-week health overhaul each year. As you can imagine, these tough individuals often wait until things are falling apart before they start to attend to their health and longevity. These warriors can and will fight through incredible odds but often fall short when it comes to pulling the race car into the pit for maintenance and refueling. The Continue Mission/Warrior Fitness Program, in essence, brings them into the shop, puts them up on a lift, and does a complete overhaul of mind and body.

It may come as no surprise that many of us non-champion nine-to-five types also fail to pay attention to our health until things go wrong. The reality is, many of us are woefully ill-educated when it comes to interpreting signals from our bodies and taking steps to address them. If I'm being honest, I used to think that people who didn't take care of their health were just lazy. Go for a walk, lift some weights, eat your veggies, drink water, and go to bed on time—it's not that hard. If you don't do it, you must have some character flaw that keeps you from doing it. You're undisciplined, and that's all there is to it.

But I was wrong.

If that were true, how do people who have preventable lifestyle diseases (type 2 diabetes, high blood pressure, cardiovascular disease, etc.) excel as students, professionals, and family and community members? If it's just a matter of getting off your ass, how do these people do well in so many other areas of life? It can't be a character flaw. It's death by a thousand cuts again. Signals from the body go unnoticed, normal begets normal, and ever so slowly we let things slide. We don't hear the signals or can't interpret them, we hear them and ignore them altogether, or we simply don't know how to respond when a signal does come through.

Check Engine Light is the culmination of my years of work with warriors, athletes, and executives as well as regular folks who just want to stay healthy and play with our kids and grandkids. Much of my career has revolved around clients who were already banged up, broken, and torn down. In the absence of obvious trauma to the body, many of the people I've worked with had no real idea what was causing their problems. As we worked together, we would uncover that small warning lights were often flickering long before the larger malfunction showed up. Unfortunately, unlike a car, your body doesn't come with an owner's manual. So, when the check engine light pops on, you can't just turn to page fifty-three and find out what it means—until now.

That's the whole enchilada with this book. I want to share with you what I've learned about listening to and working with the body to build a dashboard of reliable indicator lights that let you know when you're headed for trouble. You will also develop a toolkit so that you can do some basic maintenance on your body. Doing so helps you stay on the road to performing at your best regardless of your chosen pursuit. It's not just those who serve at the tip of the spear in the military, elite athletes, and C-suite executives who must learn to listen to the engine and watch the dashboard. We all do.

ACKNOWLEDGMENTS

Thank you to Alex Oliver of Virginia High Performance and Alison Messick of the Navy SEAL Foundation, who believed in this material in its infancy. Had I not had the opportunity to work this material out with our nation's warriors, it would have remained an analogy that lived only in my mind.

Thank you to Fremont Press for taking a chance on me, a little-known coach and health educator who thought he might have a good idea.

To my wife, Thomi: Nothing I've accomplished would have been possible without your encouragement and, at least as important, your challenge to do and be better. If not for your grace and love, I would certainly be a lesser man.

Mom: Through your actions you showed me what it means to be a teacher in the deepest sense of the word. Thanks for teaching me how to think, not what to think. Being your son has been a winning lotto ticket.

Punky: You were an awesome kid, and now you are an impressive woman. Being your dad set me on track to engage with life in a way I never expected but am eternally grateful for.

I've had lots of mentors over my twenty years in this field. Without their help and guidance, I certainly would not have amounted to much. These are just a few who have made an indelible mark on me as a person and as a human performance professional.

Kelly Starrett: You have never owed me one thing but have been incredibly generous with me since our first conversation many years ago. Thank you from the bottom of my heart for the continued friendship and guidance through the years. Your sincere encouragement has given me steam at times when it was sorely needed. It has meant more to me than you know.

The late Al Walke of Flex Gym: Flex Gym has been a mecca of bodybuilding and strength on the East Coast of the U.S. for decades, and "Big Al" was at the helm for many years. Flex was my first gym "home." Early in my life, Al stoked my interest in understanding how the human body moves. He answered endless questions from me about strength and conditioning throughout my youth, always with a warm smile and a sarcastic comment. His influence is still deep in my bones.

The late Dr. Peter Schoeb: By the time we met, Peter had probably forgotten more about anatomy, physiology, and manual therapy than I'll ever learn. Although he referred to himself as a "Swiss hillbilly," Dr. Schoeb was one of the most brilliant clinicians I've ever met. He looked to things that were tried and true and was an early example of how to marry sound scientific reasoning with a well-developed gut instinct based on experience. Like Big Al, Peter answered what I'm sure seemed like ceaseless interrogation from me.

Frank Cucci: Another man I accosted with questions. There might be a theme here. I joined Linxx Academy of Martial Arts when I was thirteen. The entirety of my teenage years were spent there, and during that time I had the opportunity to be mentored by you and the other rugged men who were a part of that culture, some of whom I am still friends with thirty years later. My time there showed me what real effort in training could get you and how the hardships that come with good, committed training could make you stronger in mind, body, and spirit. I can never repay the gifts I got from that time, but I do my best to pay it forward.

BP and JK: My first space monkeys. You started as clients and now you're my brothers. You both have had my back since way back. Thank you.

More friends and colleagues who are in my cabal and have influenced my path: Everybody at ALTIS, but especially coaches Dan Pfaff and Stu

MacMillan. The team at Virginia High Performance—special shout-out to director of programs Jacob Lonowski for mind-expanding discussions. Danny Foley of Rude Rock Strength and Conditioning—keep smiling. Danny Yeager and Kevin Kirsch—those Art of Breath days have a special place in my heart. Coach Greg Souders of Standard Jiu Jitsu—may the weekly calls about jiu-jitsu and life continue. Nestor Bayot of Coastal Brazilian Jiu Jitsu—a man who not only teaches good jiu-jitsu but also helps forge good humans. To the CrossFit community in Virginia Beach, Virginia, that sustained my work for years and the greater CrossFit Affiliate community worldwide that has provided countless opportunities for me to teach and learn, thank you for your openness and generosity. Thanks to Coach Phil Sabatini of East Coast Gold for showing me what weightlifting really is. To all of the athletes, students, clients, and mentees I've had over the years, thank you for the opportunity to fulfill my life's work. Continuing to learn along with you has elevated me as a coach and as a person.

If there's anybody I've forgotten, my bad. Don't take it personally. Or do. Just don't tell me.

INTRODUCTION

When I was growing up, I had friends, and maybe you did too, who loved to work on cars. Their family was always in the garage on the weekend with tools in their hands, turning a wrench on something, whether it was an oil change on Mom's car or fixing the brakes on a friend's truck. Then, when we got our licenses, that same friend would notice things not just about their own vehicle but about mine, too. We'd hop in to go our favorite hangout spot, turn the key, and they'd say, "Wait a second. Is your muffler tie a little loose?" I hadn't even noticed an unusual sound, and I drove the truck every day. How in the holy heck did they notice it? Super hearing? Genius mind powers? No, they were attuned to those signals from experience.

Just to be clear, I was not that kid. I wasn't the friend who knew about how to use tools or fix your car. Call somebody else for that. (Andy V., if you read this book, reach out—my tire pressure sensor needs attention.) I was, however, the fitness kid. My parents were athletes who competed at national and international levels. My mother competed in all kinds of events: bodybuilding, arm wrestling, marathon running, and even obstacle course racing. My stepfather was an accomplished martial artist. That meant I was around physical training and performance environments constantly. As a preteen, I hung out and later trained in one of the premier bodybuilding gyms on the East Coast of the United States, Flex Gym. Legendary head trainer Al Walke was a mentor of mine.

I started training in martial arts at around six years old and was lifting weights by the time I was twelve or so. In my teens, I became the "How do I get fit?" kid. I started taking friends to the local rec center to show them how to lift weights and get strong even before I could drive. While writing this book, I was catching up with a good buddy of mine whom I've known since high school. He politely listened to me explain the premise and how I was putting it together, and then he said, "Oh, so what you've always done. Just now in a book." Well, yeah.

I'm not saying all this to suggest that my anecdotal experience as a fitness and martial arts nerd qualifies me to tell you how to be healthy. Those early years, though, did inform much of the way I attune myself to information from my body. It wasn't until much later in life that I realized not everybody knows what the clicking in the engine means. I had access to unique information that was supported by long experience, on top of which I'd built an entire career in human performance. It's those insights that are built into the content I present in this book, which is a formal interpretation of hundreds, if not thousands, of conversations I have had with friends, clients, students, and other performance professionals. Check Engine Light is a convenient analogy for paying attention to your body. The more I explored it, the more the Muse spoke to me from the ether.

Check Engine Light wasn't supposed to be a book. I didn't come up with a pitch for this book and then slap together ideas in order to "get published." It started as a simple analogy that I used to get the people I work with to pay better attention to signals from their bodies. I like this analogy because it pulls out feelings of judgment that often come packaged with thinking about health, especially the things that are lacking. Just recently, I was talking to a friend about his low back seizing up, and when I asked what he'd been doing to prevent it from happening again, his answer was filled with undertones of guilt and embarrassment. I wasn't casting any judgment on him; nobody does all of the things they're supposed to do all the time. I just wanted to have a better idea of what was going on so I could help.

Another antagonistic viewpoint to appropriately managing self-care is toughness. When I work with competitive athletes (especially in combat sports) as well as professionals who need to be exceptionally resilient to do their jobs, like first responders, they often think they don't need this stuff because they're "doing just fine" without it. They might even have convinced themselves that taking care of themselves is a sign of weakness. Meanwhile, the reality is that they are often masking pain, hiding injuries, or ignoring outright illness. Check Engine Light became an easy way to communicate the idea that our bodies have ways to send warning signs to us, and if we ignore them, stuff is going to break. Just like any vehicle they drive or equipment they operate. It's as simple as that.

This analogy seemed to land especially well with the military and tactical populations I have spent much of my career working with. As time went on, the idea grew into a set of ideas, and after some time unofficially working with the team at Virginia High Performance (owned and operated by retired Navy SEAL Alex Oliver, a pioneer of human performance in special operations), I was invited to turn it into a full-blown curriculum and teach it as part of the Continue Mission/Warrior Fitness Program. That afforded me the chance to iterate the presentation and deployment of these ideas at a rate that otherwise would have taken years. As I refined this material through dialogue with the clients and professionals around me, as well as with outside groups, it occurred to me that I had something that could help anybody, regardless of their background. I should say, and I mean this in all seriousness, that the work told me it was a book.

MISSION STATEMENT

I'd like to take a little more time here to explain my mission as a coach, educator, and author. It will help clarify why I've made certain decisions about the way I present the material in the *Check Engine Light* book and workbook. Let me start with a brief story.

Nine years or so after I graduated from the Cayce/Reilly School of Massage, I was invited to come back and teach. The school was restructuring its curriculum and wanted me to write a new course. At first, they requested myofascial release and trigger point–type classes—technique-specific offerings that I had developed expertise in during my time working as a massage therapist. I said no. Instead, I offered to come teach if and only if I could develop a class on clinical reasoning. Many of the classes I took both during my time at Cayce/Reilly and after were focused on techniques and protocols, but very few taught a practitioner how to thoughtfully assess a client and execute a course of action. This bothered me because, as I had experienced, on your first day at work as a massage therapist, somebody is going to come in with pain or dysfunction and expect that you can do something to relieve it. How can this be responsibly done without a thorough and accurate assessment? It can't. So we can pour all of the techniques in the world into students, but if they aren't able to think critically about the problems that are confronting their clients, who cares?

This same exact thing is happening in the health market today. The information age has given us access to vastly more data than ever before. At the tap of a screen, or even more recently, the sound of your voice, you can have the cumulative knowledge of human history at your beck and call. But having access to all of the experts, research, podcasts, apps, and programs in the world isn't moving the needle in the right direction. In fact, it seems that we are getting sicker and sicker. So maybe information alone isn't the answer? To that end, it is my deep-seated opinion that the delivery of data is the lowest form of education we can offer. As Alexander Dumas said, "There are those who have knowledge and those who have understanding. The first requires memory and the second philosophy." Real education is forming a meaningful and personal connection with the pursuit of understanding and becoming autonomous in that pursuit.

Of course, the delivery of information and data does play a role, but it's a much smaller part than you might think. If I had to summarize my mission as a coach, practitioner, and teacher in one word, it would be *autonomy*. Above all else, I want you to develop ownership over your own process. How that expresses itself can vary greatly between individuals, no doubt, but it does not ultimately change my orientation as an educator.

I'm interested in cultivating self-determination and skill in the domain of health. I want you to be able to think critically about why things are happening, what you want, and how to pursue it. The best outcome I can think of is that the lessons you learn from this book will become such an intuitive part of your life that you'll nearly forget about this book altogether.

HOW TO READ THIS BOOK

Check Engine Light isn't just another nonfiction book about being healthy. It's an educational guidebook that you can use to explore your health and performance for a lifetime. As such, it was written to suit different learning styles and goals. There are a few ways you could read this book:

- **Cover to Cover:** You could go old school and read this book from start to finish in consecutive order. After you make it through the core material, you move on to the Personal Health Experiments outlined in the workbook.

- **Reflect and Experiment as You Go:** You can read the book straight through and, as you do, follow along in the workbook for additional reinforcement. This is the college textbook style of reading this book.

- **Pick a Patty:** This book is kind of like a triple-decker hamburger. Sections One and Three (Chapters 1 through 3 and 7 and 8, respectively) are like the buns. Section Two is like the three burger patties in the center. You can read the buns of the burger and then choose one of the patties to focus on first, working through the experiments in the workbook concurrently.

Whichever way you choose, I highly recommend reading Section One before you do anything else. Otherwise, the setup of the experiments won't make nearly as much sense.

Additionally, in each chapter there are self-reflection questions. These are not hokey quiz questions about William Shakespeare like the ones in your old SAT prep workbook. They are based on real conversations and insights I've had with clients over the years that have helped them develop autonomy over their own performance longevity process.

On a practical note: The questions are mostly in short-answer form with some space to handwrite your answers. In an ideal world, you would write the answers in a predetermined place (in the space provided or in a notebook) because writing things by hand has learning advantages over typing or not writing at all. Since we do not live in an ideal world, however, I suggest as a second option to think deeply about each question asked. Search for a real answer based on the information you learned and how it jibes with your experience. Also, talk to other people about it. Ask them what they think about the questions being posed. In other words, don't just fill it out to completion like you did with a middle school history test. There are no grades here. The only measure of success is that you deepen your understanding of your health and performance enough to become a more conscious participant in its development.

INVITATION AND THANK YOU

Rather than offer you a set of cookie-cutter solutions or rote protocols, I offer you an invitation to think critically, to practice, and to truly learn. I invite you to become your own personal health scientist—to experiment and find what works for you. You don't have to turn into a wheatgrass-drinking health nut (not that there's anything wrong with that), but it behooves all of us to be conscious participants in the evolution of our health. Everybody is forced to pay attention to their health at some point; it is just a matter of when. With that, I'd like to encourage you to immerse yourself in this lifelong endeavor.

Along with my invitation, I'd like to add a request. I ask that as you experiment and learn, you invite others along with you—to share your process with your family, friends, and community. Also, please share what you learn with me. You can find me on social media by searching @thecheckenginelight, or you can check out the weekly articles I publish at checkenginelight.substack.com. My knowledge of these topics is still growing every single day. Please offer up your own experience and insight so we can all work together toward improved health and performance.

Thanks very much for taking the time to read this book. I truly hope the ideas and practices add value to your pursuit of a healthy and meaningful life.

Rob Wilson

SECTION ONE
CALIBRATING PERCEPTION

Section 1 sets the stage for the entire book. These three chapters introduce you to some of the main ideas that drive this philosophy of performance longevity and set the stage for running successful personal health experiments.

I'll dive into why it's important to calibrate your perception of your health status and how to develop valid, reliable, and accessible indicators to do so. Also covered are key concepts such as analyzing trends and having a schema for selecting tools for your system of performance longevity.

I highly recommend using the self-reflection questions included at the end of each chapter to think through these ideas more carefully and take ownership of the concepts so that they are relevant to you and your needs.

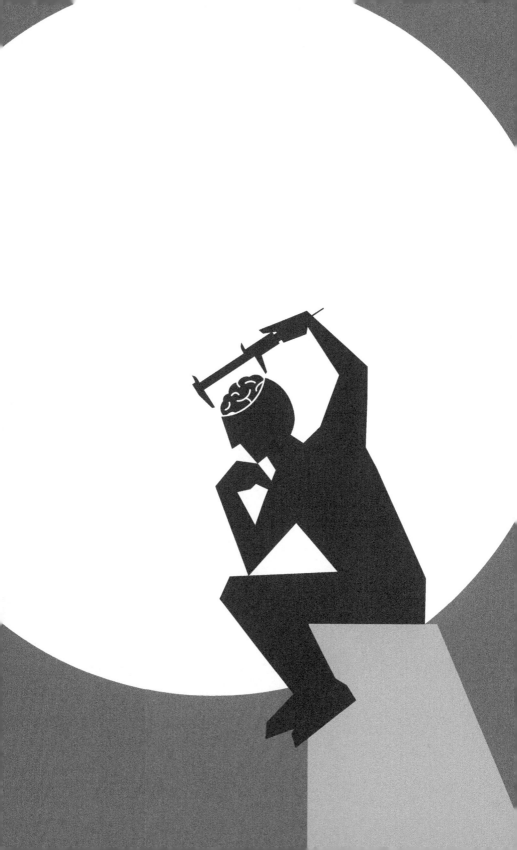

CHAPTER 1 | The Flashing Orange Light

Imagine this: You're in your car on your way to pick up Luna, your three-year-old French bulldog, from doggy daycare, and gnarly dark gray smoke begins to emanate from under the hood. With a shudder and a cough, the engine shuts down, and you have to coast into the emergency lane. A minute ago, this marvel of modern machinery was running like a top and—bam!—out of nowhere, this hunk of junk goes kaput and leaves you stranded. Now you have to call for a tow, get somebody else to pick up Luna before you get slammed with a late fee, and deal with whatever strains on your bank account are forthcoming. You smack your hands on the steering wheel and yell some obscenity to the tune of "This damn car!"

As you stare into the glare of your dashboard, something catches your eye: a little flashing orange light. The check engine light. *How long has that thing been on, anyway?* you wonder. *It kinda seems like it's always been on.* Then it dawns on you—you were supposed to take this jalopy in for service weeks ago. The light kept flashing, but between traffic and work and family obligations, you either kept forgetting or ignored it altogether. Now here you are on the side of the road, forehead glowing ever redder from the palm of your own hand smacking it. If only some flashing light in your field of vision would have alerted you before it got this bad!

These kinds of things happen all the time. I know I've seized a truck engine (or two), and it darn sure wasn't the truck's fault. There were warning signs way ahead of system failure. Some I could have handled myself and others required more savvy and expertise, but all were preventable. What's funny is that if you think about a car, truck, or really any machine, it seems pretty obvious. While these ideas seem obvious when it comes to the care of the machines we operate and the equipment we use, many of us fall short in applying these same concepts to our own self-care.

In my two-plus decades as a health and performance professional, one thing has become exceedingly clear: We are often disconnected from the things that drive our health and performance until they reach a critical mass of dysfunction—just like ignoring the check engine light in your car until the engine seizes and you're stranded on the side of the road. We beat up our bodies, neglect to give them proper attention and maintenance, and then, when systems malfunction, we blame our "bad" joints, our "weak" hearts, our "unlucky" genetics, or whatever else comes to mind rather than our own failure to care for ourselves. Of course, there are factors outside of our control that may predispose us to one type of health issue or another. There isn't much we can do about road conditions. What we can do is learn to drive skillfully, watch for indicators telling us that something requires our attention, and maintain our vehicles properly.

Small problems left unattended beget larger problems. If you don't rotate your tires, your tires wear unevenly. When your tires wear unevenly, your steering starts to pull. As your steering pulls more, your struts, shocks, and brakes wear out faster. Compensation moves its way through the whole system, and before you know it, more things seem to be going wrong than right. Now it's an additional burden to get to work and pick up the kids from school. What was once a small crack in the ice spreads throughout the whole pond. Of course, not every small problem becomes catastrophic. But the purpose of maintaining your vehicle isn't just to prevent it from break-ing down. Staying tuned in to how your vehicle is running also means it'll work if and when you need it to perform.

These same rules apply to maintaining your health and performance. Knowing when to pull over and when to keep on keeping on can be tough, though. Thankfully, your biology comes equipped with some built-in indicator lights that let you know when you are bumping into potential problems, but it's ultimately up to you to dig deeper into what they mean.

BUILT-IN BIOLOGY

Over the course of my career, I've learned that very few people are truly aware of what's going on under the hood. Even if they do have some sense of it, they often struggle to articulate it. During my tenure as a massage therapist, I had to poke, prod, cajole, and coax out more detailed descriptions of what my clients were feeling in order to determine exactly what was going on. It was not uncommon for clients to provide information that was incomplete or even outright incorrect during the assessment process, not because they were disingenuous or cagey but because they didn't have precise reference points to adequately describe their experiences. Not only that, but the human nervous system is designed primarily to consolidate information in a way that allows us to solve problems moving forward, not keep a detailed log of every experience we've ever had.

The point of any worthwhile health assessment is to clarify what the signals coming from your body are really telling you so that you can decide on a course of action, whether it's to keep doing what you're doing or make a change. If a report of discomfort was the only evidence to go on, helping people resolve their pain and movement dysfunctions would be much more difficult. When you go to the doctor a month into your new pickleball obsession because your elbow hurts so much that you can't brush your teeth, the doctor will ask you a series of questions and perform an examination. That's because "my elbow hurts" tells us only one thing for sure—that your elbow hurts. It's insufficient information from which to draw conclusions or decide how to address the deeper problem. The real who, what, when, where, why, and how have yet to be determined.

Your beautifully engineered nervous system senses and perceives information from both your external and your internal environments in order to guide your behaviors. These neurological sensations and perceptions can be categorized as exteroception and interoception, respectively.

- **Exteroception** answers the question *What's going on out there?* It includes the five senses of touch, taste, hearing, smell, and sight. Exteroception is the brain's interpretation of these sensations so you know what's going on in the outside world. The vast majority of our attention is focused on exteroception because both threats and opportunities mostly show up in the external world, at least evolutionarily speaking. High performers in particular are often highly attuned to the external environment. Not only that, but some life experiences, like careers in the military or law enforcement, can further exaggerate the natural tendency toward exteroceptive focus.

- **Interoception** answers the question *What's going on in here?* It is the collection of your internal sensations and perceptions as organized by your brain. These include physiological processes like heartbeat, breathing, and digestion and physiological sensations like pain. Interoception is your felt sense of your internal state. Psychological, emotional, and physiological cues are perceived and interpreted through the filter of your experience. This interwovenness is so seamless that physical descriptions of emotional states are part and parcel of everyday language. Phrases like "gut-wrenching anxiety," "a broken heart," and "nerves of steel" are commonly used to describe our internal states. While developing interoception is an essential part of the pursuit of health, it's important to remember that perceptions can be flawed and biased, which means they require regular calibration—a topic I'll spend some time on in the coming pages.

Most of the ways we categorize sensations from the body can be limited by overlapping functions in the indicator lights. For example, pain can result from exertion, mood changes, local inflammation, or a legitimate biomechanical insult. Just as the check engine light in a car simply means to check the engine, a biological indicator light such as pain is a prompt for further investigation.

An additional limitation is that most of us have a narrow vocabulary regarding how our bodies function. And why wouldn't we? Most of us aren't health experts with more than a rudimentary education in anatomy and physiology. However, if you have a planned, organized, and systematic approach to interfacing with your body for the purpose of maintaining its function, you'll develop more precise terms to describe how you're feeling and moving. In time, you'll be able to better differentiate sensations in your body, and if the occasion arises, you'll be able to communicate more clearly with healthcare professionals. That's one of the goals of this book: to deliver a framework for how to read the signals and either reach into your own toolbox to address it or at least have better information for the mechanic when you roll into the shop. You don't have to be able to reprogram your car's computer, but you should be able to change the tire. Catch my drift?

CAN YOU TRUST HOW YOU FEEL?

Your default internal indicators, while biologically sufficient for the purposes of survival, do not serve the more sophisticated goal of doing your best at whatever it is you wish to do for the long haul. They have some design features that make them less than optimal for helping you predict trends in your health and performance. For one, they're subjective. Moods, feelings, and perceptions can vary wildly from person to person. Pain, by way of example, gets your attention but is flawed in its subjectivity and vagueness. Chronic pain is the number one reason for doctors' visits. While we all know pain when we feel it, it's difficult to compare your own experience of pain to another person's experience and determine what is causing it for each person individually.

Furthermore, your acute psycho-emotional state and the corresponding neurological signature plays an important role in the experience of pain. In one study of burn victims, arousal (how stressed or relaxed the nervous system is) was shown to have a significant effect on the discomfort associated with the treatment of third-degree burns. Patients who felt anxious prior to treatment reported more intense pain than those who were not anxious or, in the case of this particular study, used controlled breathing techniques to reduce feelings of dread. Our internal stress levels can have real effects on our perception of pain, pleasure, and much more.

It's not always easy to interpret signals from your body. When the check engine light pops up on your dashboard, there are a host of things that could be going awry under the hood. Similarly, your physiological indicators don't offer a detailed manuscript that tells the whole story of what's going on. That's far too complicated. Our biology simply wants to send signals that shape behaviors according to our environment. Anything more sophisticated, like performance, health, or longevity, is a purely human concoction. Over time, it's essential that we learn to inform our perceptions, gut feelings, and intuitions with better-quality information. This way, you can better understand how you are feeling and performing, allowing you to respond with more precise adjustments to your behavior if you so choose.

Furthermore, your perceptions are based on what is normal for you. The human body comes equipped with a sort of set of internal thermostats. Like the thermostats in our homes trip the switch for the heat or air-conditioning to come on when the temperature hits a certain point, sensors in your body trip a switch when you hit certain points to indicate that it's time for physiological or behavioral change. While these sensory bodies have their own physiological standards for our species, within those tolerances they are further calibrated according to the behaviors you engage in and the environments you are exposed to. In other words, your experience plays an important role in how you interpret signals from your body.

For many people, it feels normal to experience chronic pain, anxiety and depression, low energy, poor mood, and lack of focus or motivation. *Normal*, though, is a word that describes frequency over time, not optimal or efficient function. Our thresholds for normal and the constituent indicators were not built with the long-term health effects of too many potato chips in mind. In fact, just the opposite. Those deep metabolic administrators are only concerned with caloric and nutrient intakes that sustain the most basic biological functions. Longer-term planning has to come from the higher-order parts of the brain that all too often are trumped by feelings, habits, and customs. This includes your relationship with the signals your body uses to communicate its needs.

THERMOSTATS AND THRESHOLDS

In what seems like the all-too-distant past, my wife and I purchased a home in Virginia Beach, Virginia. It was a rehabilitation project home that was built in 1950 and had since changed ownership several times. Through squatters, poor add-on construction, and double mortgage defaults, the property was lost to the bank, fell into some disrepair, and then landed in our care. When we moved in and for about eight years afterward, the home had no central heat or air-conditioning. None. Zero. Zilch. If you really want to test your comfort thresholds (and your marriage), try living in a house that has no A/C during a swampy 100-degree Virginia Beach summer. To make matters even more interesting, the average February high was a toasty 45 degrees—indoors. Not ideal sleeping temperatures by any means.

While contending with those temperatures was no picnic at first, eventually they hardly registered as uncomfortable. Moreover, when we went places that did have central heating and cooling, it felt…weird. During the extreme-weather times of the year, having access to climate control did sometimes come as a relief, but for the most part, we just became accustomed to going without. A major downside, however, was that dust, mold, and moisture accumulated inside our house, leading to furniture damage. No bueno, no bueno indeed. We humans can get used to damn near anything. It's both a superpower and a curse.

The point of this story is that our internal physiology comes with some clearly defined tolerances. If things stray too far outside of our homeostatic boundaries (the thresholds of stable physiological conditions in the human body—i.e., temperature, blood pressure, etc.), signals will fire off to tell us that we'd better change our behavior before things get too dodgy. For example, the pH of human blood is 7.35 to 7.45. If we start to push into either a more acidic or a more alkaline state, the body responds with a fast change in respiratory patterns to get us back into our lane. As we become less and less efficient, as it happens when we get out of shape or develop a cardiovascular or metabolic disease, our respiratory patterns start to give us clues about how well we are managing the waste products of bodily movement—not just the gym kind, but the life kind, too. What the heck does that have to do with checking engines and indicators and trusting your sense of what's going on in your body?

Everything.

As we walk down the road toward disease, dysfunction, and reduced well-being, there are often signs posted all over the place, but we just don't realize it. A tiny loss of movement capacity here and a little more breathlessness there doesn't seem like a big deal and probably won't capture our attention. We just get used to it. Just as we can expand our tolerance of stress and discomfort (such as through exercise), we can reduce it through a lack of awareness and exposure. What becomes comfortable and typical for us from day to day may not be what's best for us over the long haul—and very often isn't.

PERFORMANCE LONGEVITY

All of this can't just be about avoiding disease, injury, and dysfunction. What is it that we're really striving for? The topic of the day is longevity, lifespan, health span, or whatever label you want to put on it. While, as a person in the autumn of life, I do have an appreciation for these ideas, they don't really speak to a motivation that will drive us to sustain the habits necessary for not only avoiding that which we don't want but more so moving toward what we do want. I want to know that every morning when I get in my truck and turn the key, the engine is going to fire. Not only that, but I want a reliable vehicle that will get me and my family where we need to go. I want my truck to be able to pull trailers and haul furniture. I want my truck to be able to drive long distances and get my wife to the hospital in an emergency. I want my truck to not only not break down, but to perform. Not just today, but for as long as possible. The way to achieve that? Regular maintenance, repairs when necessary, and upgrades as needed or desired.

The same goes true for what you want from your body and mind. Do you really want to hang on a thread just below the threshold for the emergency bells ringing? Or do you want the feeling of knowing that you can execute when you want to, how you want to?

Our goal, then, is what I've come to call performance longevity. Performance is about execution. Can you do *the thing*? What is the thing? It's whatever you care about, whatever is important to you. For the tactical professionals I work with, performance means the ability to execute under the deeply strenuous demands of a career in the military, law enforcement, or emergency services. For you, it might mean doing the best you can at your job, or as a parent or spouse. Performance for you might mean being able to maintain and enjoy your hobbies, or maybe it means picking up your grandkids. It will mean different things to different people at different times in life. What stays the same is that performance means execution. Longevity means duration of life. So what's the shelf life of your performance? How long will you be able to execute?

Will you last longer if you pay attention to how your vehicle is running, perform proper maintenance, and make adjustments when necessary? Or if you wait until the oil runs dry, ignore warning signals, and drive like nothing is happening? Maybe you own a really robust, well-made vehicle. That's great. Some are made a little stronger than others. It's a nice safety net when it's not possible to pull into the shop. But if you want that robustness to last, proper care is essential.

All of this is as true of your body and mind as it is for anything else that you want to extract value from in life. If you invest in those things with care, you compound your returns. If you ignore them, you accrue debt.

While the automotive analogy is one that helps you more clearly understand what happens if you fail to address issues, there is a key difference. If you don't take care of your car, you can get a new one. You have but one body. You are stuck with the consequences of your "driving" for life. It behooves you, then, to become a better driver of body and mind. You are obligated to know the basics of your own maintenance. Learning to properly tune yourself so that you can fire on all cylinders for as long as possible is potentially the most important skill set that a person can develop.

Although health and biology are far more complex than any automobile, caring for them doesn't have to be complicated. In the coming pages, I am going to outline a concise framework that will help you learn to pay attention to your body by showing you how to build a Performance Longevity Dashboard made of key performance indicators. This will help you continually calibrate your perception of your internal state over time so that you can use your indicators to become a better driver. You'll learn to build a toolkit as well so that you can address issues when gauges on the dashboard get your attention. Ultimately, you will gain skills that help you tune your body and mind so that all of the component parts that influence performance longevity can work in harmony to help you feel and perform your best for as long as possible.

A BETTER SYSTEM

Our internal perceptions of our state of being can be unreliable, vague, and subjective. To calibrate your perception, it helps to build some kind of system that illuminates your physiological sensitivities and helps you interpret and clarify the signals your body is sending. Just as the dashboard in your car lets you know how hard your engine is working and how fast you're driving, you can build a dashboard of indicators that give you insight into your health and performance. This way, you'll know not just how well your body is running at the moment, but also how you can expect it to run if you keep things up.

In order to do that, you need reliable indicators that give you insight into what's going on under the hood so you can make a fair assessment of your health and performance. This way, you can get ahead of the curve and address small problems before they snowball into bigger ones. Your perceptions of how you're thinking, feeling, and performing are important because they represent the voice inside. Those perceptions work best when filtered through an intelligent feedback loop that serves you over the long term. This system or practice does not need to be complicated or burdensome to use. There are many ways to take stock of what's going on inside. It can be as sophisticated as using technology to track and record markers on a regular basis or as nondescript as paying clear attention to daily habits and behaviors. In my experience, there is an elegant middle ground that allows us to take advantage of the precision of using technology to gather data while building practices that are easy to implement into our everyday lives.

SELF-REFLECTION QUESTIONS

Before you move on to Chapter 2, take some time to ask yourself these questions and reflect on your answers. I encourage you to grab a notebook or your laptop and write those answers down if you're so inclined.

Can you think of a time when you were forced to ignore a warning light from your body? What was it?

Why did you ignore it?

Did you get back to it later? If so, what did you do?

If you didn't get back to it later, why not? And what were the consequences?

_____

_____

Some cars, trucks, and even motorcycles have a feature called Limp Mode. When the vehicle's computer detects faults in critical systems, like faulty sensors, transmission issues, or low fluid levels, this security feature reduces RPMs and even shuts off nonessential functions like the radio and air-conditioning. Can you think of a time that your body went into Limp Mode?

_____

_____

> **"**It's not what you look at that matters; it's what you see.**"**
>
> —Henry David Thoreau

CHAPTER 2: | Indicators and Dashboards

C alibrating your internal perceptions requires you to become conscious of the inner workings of your body and mind and to measure and track them to some degree. While degrees of precision may vary, what is important is to have valid, reliable, and accessible indicators that provide you with information so that you can make adjustments to the way you drive and care for the vehicle of life you inhabit. Collecting these indicators can help you stay aware of what is going on in the deeper layers of your mind and body. Additionally, learning how those components interact to produce the way you're feeling at any given time can also help you predict with more certainty what problems and/or opportunities might arise in the future.

The Occupational Safety and Health Administration (OSHA) is responsible for "ensuring safe and healthful working conditions for workers by setting and enforcing standards and by providing training, outreach, education and assistance." This organization writes and enforces workplace safety regulations and conducts studies about best practices in workplace injury prevention. OSHA looks into everything from back injury statistics in hospital personnel to equipment maintenance and operation on construction sites. They're the people who mandate the signs reminding you to wear your hard hat and put away your tools. When OSHA audits a workplace, the inspectors perform an analysis of what kind of and how many workplace safety incidents are occurring, at what frequency, and how they can be reduced and prevented in the future.

When analyzing best practices in large, complex systems like hospital and construction safety, it is easy to get overwhelmed by the sheer volume of factors to consider when trying to prevent errors—especially errors that can lead not only to losses in efficiency but potentially to loss of life and limb. Looking at every tiny detail is just not possible. So what can be done to manage all of that information and create meaningful processes of improvement?

One of the ways organizations like OSHA manage complex problems is by using a system of key performance indicators. Key performance indicators, or KPIs, are metrics that inform us how close we are to achieving a certain standard, goal, or target. We use KPIs to identify the most important bits of information that we need to direct our attention to in order to get a sense of the big picture without getting lost in minutiae. This encourages us to stay on track if we're headed down the right path or course-correct if we're headed down the wrong one.

Key performance indicators aren't just used by OSHA, either. You'll find them everywhere in industry, business, coaching, and medicine. If you think about it for a minute, you'll even find that you've chosen some kind of signal to let you know if you're on track toward a goal, even if you don't think of it explicitly as a KPI. It's a natural thing to do when you create a goal. If you've ever saved coins in a jar, seeing how full that jar is every month is a KPI of how your savings plan is going. That's fine for savings that will add up to spending money for a vacation or a new air fryer, but it may be wise to be a bit more sophisticated when it comes to tracking our health and performance.

Building a set of KPIs is essential for managing our health because we can easily be tricked by our own perceptions. Our biology is incredibly complex and primarily oriented on navigating our external environment. This often causes subtle cues from the body and brain to get lost in the noise. KPIs give us markers that cue our attention so we can become more aware of changes and patterns inside the body. They provide vital signs that are valid, reliable, and (should) make sense to us.

So how do we use key performance indicators to inform our built-in, intuitive perceptions of our health and performance? How does this improved access to data lead to measurable improvements in performance longevity?

I'm glad you asked.

SELF-REFLECTION QUESTIONS

List a few examples of KPIs that you use in your life. They could be anything from indicators you use in your family to determine your kids' allowance, KPIs used at work to track progress, or even markers you use to maintain your home or automobile.

_____

_____

How do these KPIs reflect what you are trying to accomplish? Think carefully.

_____

_____

Key Performance Questions: A Prerequisite to KPIs

Before you identify your KPIs and build a health system around them, you need to establish some basic parameters to help you decide what indicators you should use. These three key performance *questions* can help you do so:

- *What do I want to achieve?* Before beginning to use KPIs, it's important to have a clear sense of what outcome(s) you want. Your answer doesn't have to be perfect or permanent, but if you have no destination, it's much harder to measure your progress.

- *What indicator(s) will let me know whether I'm on my way to that outcome or not?* When it comes to health and performance, it's hard to know what to go after and why. Make sure you understand the connection between the indicator and the outcome.

- *How will I capture this information so I can think about it later?* Whether it's as sophisticated as modern wearable gadgetry or as simple as a marker on a calendar, be certain you have a way to grab information consistently.

The process of asking and answering these questions happens over and over again in a never-ending cycle of measuring and altering the factors that influence your performance longevity. Using KPIs is much more like collecting clues to solve a mystery than it is like looking into a crystal ball. As you practice, you will develop a better sense of your personal health indicators. Revisit these questions to be sure you're paying attention to the things that truly matter.

TYPES OF KEY PERFORMANCE INDICATORS

So we've established that you need KPIs in order to have better clarity about what signals and patterns from the body to pay attention to. Now, we need to look a little deeper at the two types of KPIs: lagging indicators and leading indicators. Understanding the difference is key to staying ahead in the performance longevity game. Let's define each and then look at some case studies of how they are used.

Lagging Indicators

Lagging indicators are measurements of outcome. They're metrics that confirm whether a change has occurred and if that change was the one you were after. They answer the question: *What happened?* They're the rearview mirror. Lagging indicators can be positive, like reaching a weight loss goal, or more troublesome, like waiting to be diagnosed with diabetes before you make lifestyle changes.

Lagging indicators are important because they enable you to measure the impact of the processes you put in place (whether you did so consciously or not). In business, for example, year-end profits are an important lagging indicator about the health of a company based on the previous year's policies, actions, and processes. The amount of money the business made that year is important to know, but it's not the whole picture. If you want to repeat good outcomes or avoid bad ones, you need insight into the processes used along the way. That comes in the form of leading indicators.

SELF-REFLECTION QUESTIONS

What's an example of a lagging indicator that has shown up in your life?

_____

_____

How did you respond to that indicator?

_____

_____

What resulted as a response?

_____

_____

Leading Indicators

Leading indicators give you insight into process. They let you know if you're going in the right direction. If lagging indicators are the rearview mirror, leading indicators are the windshield. They answer the question: *Am I on the way?* Or, perhaps more precisely, *What am I on the way to?* To stick with the diabetes example, the biomarker hemoglobin A1C, which provides a snapshot of glucose in the bloodstream, is used as a leading indicator for metabolic issues that cause type 2 diabetes.

Businesses use leading indicators in conjunction with lagging indicators to get a better read on what's coming down the pipeline. For example, metrics that explain changes in costs, new customer acquisition, and customer retention are broken down in financial reports quarterly and even monthly. While leading indicators don't necessarily tell you what *will* happen, they can help you predict with more certainty what *might* happen. Ignoring the oil pressure light for three years doesn't mean your engine *will* seize, but not changing the oil certainly makes engine failure more likely.

A leading indicator that I use in my own performance longevity practice is the toe touch or forward bend found at the beginning of Sun Salutation from Hatha yoga. I have a history of low back pain and stiffness. From years of experience, I've connected loss of range of motion in the forward bend to increasing potential for back problems. Rather than waiting for my back to lock up and take me away from doing the things I love (lagging indicator), I can monitor the KPI of the toe touch so I can keep my flexibility within a certain range and even improve my capability over time.

Leading and lagging indicators probably seem familiar, even intuitive once you read about them. That's because we use them all the time to predict what might happen in the future and to measure the effects of a decision or plan. Unfortunately, we often fail to use this same logical framework with appropriate precision when it comes to behaving in ways that support performance longevity.

Let's take a deeper look at how leading and lagging indicators can play out in the real world.

What's an example of a leading indicator that has shown up in your life?

How did you respond to that indicator?

What resulted as a response?

MAKE MONEY MONEY

Key performance indicators are used everywhere. It's especially important to have a clear understanding of indicators in situations where things going wrong can have a large-scale impact. For example, the health of a national economy. Economists in governmental organizations like the Department of Commerce and the Census Bureau, private financial institutions, and wealth management conglomerates all use leading and lagging indicators to track market behavior so they can make decisions about how to move money. Both leading and lagging indicators play integral roles in both predicting economic activity and learning from upturns and downturns in markets.

Leading indicators like stock market performance, manufacturing activity, retail sales, housing prices, and new startups are used as a reflection of where the economy is headed. Retail sales are a particularly strong leading indicator because they're closely tied to manufacturing and gross domestic product. As you might imagine, when life is going well enough for people to spend money on retail goods and services (barring that it's not just an accumulation of steep debt, of course), there's a ripple effect. More goods are made, businesses hire additional employees, and the money that those new employees make goes back into the economy. While this alone is not enough to predict a bull market (when stock prices go up), it is a strong leading indicator of economic health.

Conversely, wages, unemployment rates, and gross domestic product (GDP) are lagging indicators that economists use to mark the health of the economy. These measures are slightly behind the market. They reflect how the last quarterly or yearly cycle has performed. When economic and financial think tanks are analyzing the various signs and signals of vitality, it is important to note a few key points. First, they don't use one signpost to rule them all. There are multiple points of reference that help triangulate the real processes and outcomes at play. Second, both leading and lagging indicators are used in tandem to develop a system of prediction and reflection that provides a deeper and more well-rounded perspective.

Lastly, no indicator, however seemingly reliable, is without shortcomings. Therefore, a system of multiple indicators is needed to get the best picture possible. For these reasons, it's important to regularly evaluate these indicators over time and their relevance to the bigger picture. Different components of complex systems work on different timelines, and our biology is no different.

In other words, if we want the big picture, we have to go meta. That's where trends come in.

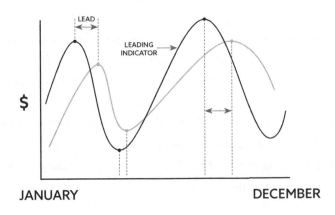

#TRENDING

As you begin to pay more attention to key performance indicators from your body, you can start to identify trends. Trends are patterns that emerge over time. Looking at trends gives you a broader perspective on the direction things are headed. Trend analysis is common practice in business, economics, and medicine. It's a reliable way to look at large sample sizes of information to identify patterns in behavior. Looking at trends takes into account the relationship between behavior, what happened before, what's happening now, and how that information can be used to more accurately predict what might be on the way.

Wearables like smartwatches use machine learning to analyze trends in the indicators embedded in their proprietary algorithms. Some smartwatches keep track of your heart rate, step count, etc., and let you know whether you're on track to your target and how you're performing over a given day, week, month, or quarter. If your watch notices a downward trend in your activity, it might sound an alert that says, "Hey there, you didn't hit your target for steps in the last 5 out of 10 days. Get moving!" The downward trend in your step count during that time period signals the software to notify you that you're moving away from your target of activity. Herein lies one of the great upsides of direct-to-consumer health wearable technology: You can catch the beginnings of trends toward things you might not want a little earlier and be encouraged to keep going when you're on the right track.

If you decide to do something different as a result of noticing a trend in behavior, health, or performance, check in with your indicators to make sure you have good information connected to your long-term outcome. Some people relish the opportunity to crunch numbers and extrapolate deep meaning from spreadsheets, graphs, and charts, but it's not necessary to get that fine-toothed to benefit from noticing trends. If you are mathematically inclined, you can go deep into the numbers. If you're not a numbers or gadget type of person, don't despair. Understanding a few fundamental properties of looking at trends can help you be more thoughtful about how you observe your internal indicators and connect them to your behavior.

A couple of things to keep in mind when you look at trends (whether through the lens of your own perception or when reading a report from your smartphone):

- **Think about why the trend occurred.** Perhaps you have missed your step goal for the past 5 days, but you were consistent for 125 days before that. Then you got sick, and your car went into the shop unexpectedly. Well, then by golly you had a good reason to downtrend. But you also noticed that without getting as much exercise, you had less energy and your sleep was a bit off. Now, the question is: How will you use this information to drive your planning moving forward? Many times, just recognizing the trend is enough to push us in the direction of getting back on the horse.

- **Make sure there are enough reference points to indicate a true trend over a given time period.** If one Instagram influencer is wearing a new style of jeans, it doesn't necessarily mean a lot. But if 50 percent of her 1.2 million followers started wearing the same jeans within a few days' time, along with using the hashtag #momjeans, now they're "trending." When you start looking at health trends through the same type of lens, it's important to make sure your sample size in a given time period indicates meaningful momentum. If you do take notice of a pattern in health emerging, be sure not to go full Chicken Little (or Henny Penny if you happen to be in Europe) without due consideration of whether what you've noticed truly indicates a trend or if you're just having an isolated experience. If you're tracking your sleep, for example, a few nights of reduced sleep quality doesn't mean you have a sleep "problem" per se. You are trending downward for all intents and purposes, but if it's a reasonable response to life demands and you climb back to normal without much fuss, you may not need to pull the fire alarm just yet. How do you know whether the trend is worthy of more attention or not? Experience is the best teacher. As Kierkegaard said, "Life can only be understood backwards; but it must be lived forwards."

Paying attention to trends allows you to better understand your patterns in health behavior so you can make more thoughtful and informed choices. It brings things that might normally slip below the radar into your conscious awareness so you can course-correct before things get too far off track. This is essential for carving an effective path toward performance longevity.

SELF-REFLECTION QUESTIONS

What personal health or performance-related trends have you ignored that resulted in negative outcomes?

_____

_____

What personal health or performance-related trends have you noticed that preceded positive outcomes?

_____

_____

BUYER BEWARE

Now that you've bought into the idea of key performance indicators, I'm going to temper that belief with some cautionary tales. While KPIs are essential for tracking progress, they aren't without flaws. KPIs have some shortcomings that can lead you astray if you don't know what to look for. Sometimes metrics come with unintended consequences, especially when you mix up your goals with your indicators. I've seen this a lot in my long career as a strength and conditioning coach. Coaches and athletes get fixated on numbers in the gym and forget that those numbers are indicators for predicting athlete robustness. Obsessing over hitting certain numbers in the gym can sometimes be to the detriment of on-field performance. These fallacies happen quite often and in all sorts of places in the domain of health and performance. Let's take a quick look at some of the ways in which the use of indicators can go wrong.

Goodhart's Law, Performance, and Effectiveness

Goodhart's Law states, "Once a measure becomes a target, it ceases to be a good measure." In other words, when you have an indicator for a particular outcome you want, and that indicator becomes the be-all, end-all in and of itself, you set yourself up for some problems.

A clear example of this concept is in the game of search engine optimization. Ever notice when using the great and powerful Google that the meat and potatoes of what you're looking for doesn't seem to come to the top of the page or even land on the first page of search results? That's partially because the "relevance" algorithm scores web pages according to indicators like keywords and link titles. The result is a constant cat-and-mouse game between the search engine companies who closely guard the purity of their algorithms and the SEO experts who game the system with facades like artificial links and keyword spamming. They find the indicator (keywords) and make it the target. Now it's no longer a good measure of the page's true relevance, so your search for a set of earplugs lands you on a page that makes you blush and delete your browser history with the record-breaking speed of a high school freshman.

There is no shortage of examples of Goodhart's Law in action; COVID-19 death count (both over- and undercounting depending on the situation), fitness tests, and even enemy combatant body counts in war. Yep, even in war. During the very unpopular Vietnam War, Defense Secretary Robert McNamara wanted to demonstrate American progress, so he used enemy body count as a measure of that progress. As you might imagine, incentivizing body count as a measure of success had some negative downstream consequences—not the least of which was Operation Speedy Express, which resulted in an estimated 5,000 civilian casualties that were often counted as enemy combatants.

Aside from that campaign, there's evidence of other bloated reports of enemy casualties. For example, the U.S. Army reported over 10,000 dead and just under 3,000 captured, but with a mere 800 weapons recovered. Perhaps the fog of war, the destruction of weapons, and the work of magic AK-47-stealing fairies can account for this disparity, but it's more likely that the numbers were fudged to make Daddy Warbucks happy. Any time we reward a measure, we have to watch out for our own insidiousness. As the saying goes, "If you ain't cheating, you ain't trying."

Often, when Goodhart's Law goes into action, measures are corrupted either by purposeful human manipulation or by pure force of situation. One way to safeguard yourself against this problem is to understand the difference between measures of performance (MOPs) and measures of effectiveness (MOEs):

- **Measures of performance** answer the questions: *Am I accomplishing the task? Did I do the right thing?*

- **Measures of effectiveness** answer the questions: *Am I creating the desired effect in the environment? Did I do the thing right?*

Human beings tune into performance outcomes quite easily. They're easier to see and measure. Measures of effectiveness can be subtler and harder to measure. One distinct example of how the two work together along with Goodhart's Law in health is weight loss.

According to the United States Centers for Disease Control, in 2022, 41.9 percent of Americans were obese. Obesity is defined as an excess of adiposity (body fat) per unit mass. Men are considered obese at above 25 percent body fat and women above 30 percent body fat. Obesity is strongly correlated with an increase in many sources of disease, discomfort, and physiological strain and dysfunction. If a person is obese and experiencing negative health consequences as a result, weight loss is probably a good option, especially if the weight lost is in the form of body fat.

Due to increasing obesity in the U.S. population, there is no shortage of diets and exercise plans that target weight loss—some good, some not so good, and some that downright push us further away from the real target:

better health. Lots of fad diets use meal replacements and appetite suppression to induce rapid weight loss. By our original measure, that will technically take a person from obese to not obese. Caloric restriction as a rule leads to weight loss, and severe caloric restriction will for all intents and purposes cause rapid weight loss. However, in so doing, we can sacrifice health at the altar of weight loss. Extreme diets are stressful on the body and can disrupt hormonal and metabolic balance. Not to mention they have proven over and over to be unsustainable and often result in a rebound effect to excessive weight gain. In many cases, the weight gained may even put the person in a worse position than when they started, with a reduced faith in weight loss programs altogether. This yo-yo effect creates a negative relationship with food and nutrition and can contribute to poor internal dialogue that in effect spirals the person further and further from the original intent.

In this example, weight loss is the measure of performance. Did you lose weight? Yes or no? For MOPs, the outcome is all that matters. The measure of effectiveness is the type of diet chosen. Did you get the desired effect? If you lost weight but ended up less healthy than when you started, you missed the point.

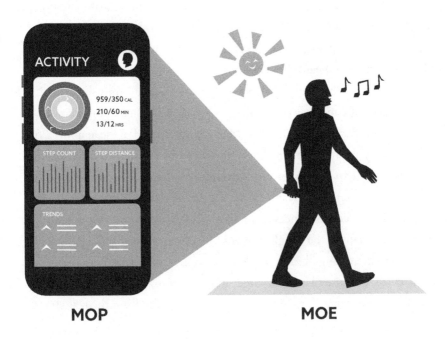

MOP   MOE

Beware the Data Trap

While it is essential to include data in your overall health schematic, however granular or broad, it comes with a bit of a warning label. Modern technology has given rise to a hyperfocus on data collection. The battle cry "Data is king" is a fantastic example of how business, healthcare, and even something as seemingly innocuous as entertainment behavior are captured, analyzed, and stored. This trend has moved its way quickly through both sports performance optimization and healthcare circles. On one hand, more reliable and valid indicators are important for describing the mechanisms underlying aspects of health. The tracking of sleep and heart rate variability are two common examples. On the other hand, too much focus on data can not only cause you to mistake the forest for the trees, but can lead to a kind of performance neurosis (broadly speaking), especially in those who may be more vulnerable. Let me provide an example.

I had an executive client for years who was deeply committed to health and performance. This person was as disciplined and steadfast as anybody I've ever worked with, and it showed both in the gym and in the board-room. They loved getting into the nitty-gritty like heart rate variability (HRV), food tracking, and regular blood work—all great indicators in their own right. We concocted an experiment to measure HRV (a reliable marker of training recovery) and sleep for between one and three months. There was regular sharing and analysis of data, and it was interesting to watch the crests and troughs in response to life and training. We learned a lot, but one lesson in particular sticks out to this day. About a month or so into the process, my client reported a consistent dip in HRV that lasted multiple days. Concurrently, they felt a bit more physically tired than normal. They couldn't seem to decipher why, and it really bothered them. *Why was I not optimized on those days? Do I need to be concerned? Should I train hard? At all?* Sleep was on point. Diet was tailored to blood work. Even accounting for intense work hours, family and work life were well organized.

When we started digging into the numbers a bit more, a couple of things became apparent. First, there really was a predictable and severe dip in HRV and readiness beginning Tuesday night and recovering to somewhat normal by Friday. After some sussing out, the issue became clearer. The cause of this dreadful lapse in optimization? Heavy deadlift sessions on Tuesday mornings. Heavy deadlifts are very stressful to the nervous system, and purposefully so. That's why they elicit such a powerful strength outcome. What we were seeing was an appropriate reaction to a potent exercise stimulus. What was more important than the HRV score each morning was the contextual information around it and what it meant for the larger picture. We wanted that reaction from the deadlifts so the body was forced to adapt to the exercise. The real questions are: How long does the return to baseline take? Is it the same each week? What confounding factors (like changes in work, family, sleep, and food) might alter those conditions? Are the readings consistent over weeks? Months? Years? What we ultimately decided to do was to move heavy deadlifts to a different day so my client would have the weekend to recover. While the stimulus and the response to that stimulus were appropriate for the situation, they contributed negatively to the flow of the week.

This particular client isn't the only person who gets fixated on the data. Basing long-term decisions on very short-term data without context is a fallacy, and unfortunately it's one that the health data industry perpetuates at times. Looking only at the types of scores that wearable devices give us for day-to-day activity can encourage shortsightedness that may direct us toward interfering too much in a natural process. Data points are like pixelations on a screen. Shoving our faces up against the screen to get a look at the individual pixels doesn't improve our viewing experience. On the contrary, in order to really see what's going on, we have to stand back a bit.

Once I started studying these concepts, I could see these issues everywhere. They sculpted the way I looked at all kinds of information, and that includes the measuring sticks I rely on in my own perceptions and biases. I promise you, as you continue on through the rest of this book and see how these ideas are illustrated in your health practice, you'll notice them everywhere. At least I did. They helped me understand how lots of systems function and malfunction, not least of which are the markers I use to track my own well-being. As we continue, we will explore specific examples of indicators, how to use them, and how to audit and recalibrate your KPIs to get the most reliable information possible.

We need indicator lights that get our attention and let us know when things are slipping so that we can start to alleviate small problems while they're still small. We need a system that lets us know what's going on and where things are headed. That system has to help us calibrate our internal perceptions and give us better information to act on. At a minimum, the system we use should inform our intuitive indicators so that when a warning light starts blinking, we have a better sense of what it means. A more systematic approach keeps us from relying too much on lagging indicators that often show up too late, or at least later than would be helpful. Our personal indicator system should help us better understand what is going on inside of us and where things are headed if we don't start to course-correct when needed.

If you've had blood work, talked to a doctor, or listened to the latest performance or longevity podcast, you know that there's no shortage of known indicators, biomarkers, and measurements for the human body. But how the heck are we supposed to organize all of that information? How do we know which markers to pay attention to and when? What we need is a simple way to group indicators so that we can take a systematic approach to knowing what's going on under the hood and what to do when things seem like they're going off track. And we need something that will help us do all this while we're driving. What we need is a dashboard.

FROM HORSE DIRT TO SPACE TRAVEL: GAUGING FUNCTION

"All models are wrong. But some are useful."

—**George R. Box**

Ever wonder where the term *dashboard* came from? When you get in your car and look over the steering wheel, you realize it's not really a board, is it? And where are the dashes? In modern transportation lingo, the dashboard is technically referred to as the "instrument cluster" or "instrument panel." Originally, the "dashboard" was a literal wooden board placed across the front of a carriage or sleigh to prevent the dirt and debris (known as dashes) kicked up by the horses from landing on the driver. Later, when the horse-less carriage arrived, the board was kept to serve a similar purpose, and then later still to protect the driver from the heat and oil that would spatter from the engine.

As automobiles evolved in sophistication, it became necessary to employ the use of gauges to monitor the vehicle's behavior. Where better to place these gauges than on the board that was already in place? As the automobile revolution took over in the twentieth century, the panel started to include safety features like padding as well as additional gauges and controls for modern functions such as heating, air-conditioning, defrosting, and of course the radio. This concept made its way across the transportation industry and was adapted for air, water, and even space travel. It's easy to imagine a pilot sitting in the cockpit of a passenger jet or a ship's helmsman standing at the wheel surrounded by the gauges and lights that help them operate their vessels.

Just as drivers, pilots, and skippers use these instrument panels to get key information about what's going on inside their machines, you too can develop a dashboard to get important information about what's going on inside the biological machine you operate every day.

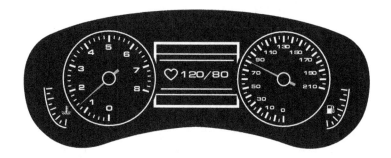

Dashboards have also made their way into computer technology and specifically data analytics. In this context, dashboards serve as a way to visually interpret large sets of data and often include key performance indicators depicted as colorful graphs and charts. Dashboards take vast amounts of technical data and distill them to those components needed for making decisions and taking action. For example, the digital dashboard on your smartphone has indicators for things like battery life, open apps, and screen time, as well as access to basic controls such as screen brightness, volume, and signal modes like airplane, Wi-Fi, and Bluetooth. There are ways to get more granular with your settings, but a quick swipe to the dashboard gives you access to the information you're most likely to need to operate the device efficiently.

Whether it's instrument panels for various forms of transportation or a visual tool for analyzing data, all dashboards have a clearly defined job: to take a lot of information from a complex system and boil it down into something that's easily implementable. That's exactly what you're going to do with the dashboard you build for performance longevity: take the plethora of information coming from the complex biological machinery of your body and whittle it down into a simple, clear, and usable format so you can more successfully pilot your body and mind. You need a dashboard composed of reliable, valid, and regular indicators that provide critical information to ensure performance longevity of the human vehicle. I call it the Performance Longevity Dashboard.

WHAT'S YOUR STATUS?

Your Performance Longevity Dashboard serves as a home base of sorts for your chosen key performance indicators. You want to use KPIs that are valid, reliable, and accessible. The validity of a measurement, in this case the KPI on your dashboard, refers to whether or not that measurement or tool is a true and accurate reflection of the thing being measured. Reliability is a measure of the consistency of a measurement within an indicator's tolerances. Accessibility means that you can physically possess the thing (obviously), but also that *you understand what the information means.*

An easy example of how these factors play out is in the use of wearables to estimate heart rate. Wrist-worn wearables are notoriously inaccurate for measuring heart rate unless they are coupled with a chest strap (although they're getting better). In other words, they don't have high validity compared to a heart rate monitor you'd get hooked up to in a hospital. But if you are wearing the same Apple Watch every day, you're probably getting pretty reliable data, meaning the watch is functioning within reasonable similar conditions from day to day. Lastly, it's accessible as long as you're wearing it and you understand how to read the information and make meaningful decisions.

Think for a moment about the dashboard in a car. Imagine all of the different gauges and indicator lights. You might think of gauges like fuel and oil pressure, temperature, and the speedometer. All of these are measures of what's going on in the automobile right now. You might also picture warning lights such as traction control, air bag, tire pressure, and, of course, the check engine light. These are indicators that something may need maintenance or repair. While the human body is vastly more complex than the simple set of indicators found in a car, or even in an aircraft, it's important to know that indicators provide information about the current condition of the body and mind, and some are warnings about where things might end up in the future if we don't course-correct.

While your Performance Longevity Dashboard may not necessarily occupy a physical space or be explicitly accessible like your car's instrument panel or the charts, graphs, and symbols commonly found in modern software, learning the underlying why of a dashboard can help you make better use of the information you receive both from and about your body and mind. Your Performance Longevity Dashboard can be comprised of a variety of indicators. They can be gauges of psychological and emotional state, energy levels and perceived stress, pain, range of motion, or even more granular physiological metrics like heart rate and blood pressure. We'll study different examples of indicators soon, but for now, what's important to know is that whatever indicators you choose should help you gain a better sense of what is happening internally (improving interoception) and provide some measurement of change if you decide to alter your course. Essentially, your dashboard helps you improve your bodily situational awareness.

In his book *Information Dashboard Design*, Stephen Few states that situational awareness works on three levels:

- Perception of the elements in the environment

- Comprehension of the current situation

- Perception of future status

In other words, do you know how your "car" is really running? What information are you using to come to that conclusion? What does your current state tell you about how your car is going to run if you continue to operate it in its current condition? At the risk of being redundant, the process of becoming more aware and acting earlier (with hopefully more accurate information) is a major part of improving performance longevity.

With all of that said, your dashboard does not need to be overly complicated. It isn't necessary for you to have the same depth of understanding of the indicators on your dashboard as health and performance professionals like doctors, nurses, dietitians, and coaches do—just like you don't need to know the same nuances of your car as the engineers who designed and built the vehicle or the mechanics who might repair it in order to be a good driver. You should, however, know what the gauges mean and, if warning lights do come on, be able to identify problems and take steps to solve them. If you get stuck, you can always get help from professionals with specialized knowledge, like doctors, physical therapists, or coaches. In the coming chapters, we are going to study specific types of indicators that you can use on your Performance Longevity Dashboard. Some are very precise physiological metrics and others are more intuitive in nature. You won't just be reading about them, either. In the workbook, I've devised ways for you to try out different indicators so you can explore what works best for you.

THE THREE FUNCTIONS OF THE PERFORMANCE LONGEVITY DASHBOARD

Let's briefly revisit some of the central concepts from earlier in this chapter. Consolidating the information will enable you to build a solid dashboard that not only will help you in the short term but will stand on solid enough ground that it can evolve with you as your understanding improves over time.

As explained previously, the purpose of key performance indicators (KPIs) is to highlight and quantify important information so you can keep track of your progress toward particular targets and goals. I also talked about types of KPIs, specifically leading and lagging indicators, which are measures of processes and outcomes, respectively. Over time, you can use leading indicators to determine if you're headed in the right direction and lagging indicators to measure the outcomes of your decisions—specifically, if you have achieved what you set out to do.

A Performance Longevity Dashboard has three foundational functions that neatly compress all of these ideas for easy reference. As you dive deeper into specific health indicators, these functions will help you stay organized and on task. Let's briefly examine each one along with a brief anecdote that highlights how it might look in real life.

It should bring clarity to problems and help you define outcomes.

If you don't know what problem you are trying to solve or what target you are trying to hit, it is difficult to plot a course and track your progress. Furthermore, the more specific you are about what it is you're after, the more precise you can be when choosing your tools, tactics, and paths. This first precept is directly connected to our earlier discussion of key performance indicators. It's important to know what it is you want to achieve and select KPIs that are directly related to the problem you are trying to solve or the target you want to hit. Sometimes that's obvious and easy and sometimes not so much.

Let's say you've got some stubborn elbow-itis from pickleball that the normal cocktail of naproxen, ice, and compression just can't seem to relieve, so you go to your trusted medical practitioner. When they see you, do they immediately reach into the medicine cabinet and give you a jar of pickleball elbow-itis relief pills? Of course not. They begin by asking you a series of questions. Then they may perform a physical exam, and based on those findings may even decide that further clarity is required, leading to an X-ray or MRI. If you get a second opinion? They'll do it all over again. Why this exhaustive and redundant process? To clarify the problem at hand. It's difficult to plan a course of action if you are unsure what it is you are dealing with in the first place. Does your elbow really hurt because of pickleball, or do you have elbow cancer that just happened to show up at the same time? Assess, don't guess.

As your care continues, your doctor or physical therapist will identify key performance indicators to mark your progress toward release from care. Resolution of pain, reduction in swelling, and ability to properly execute specific exercises all give your healthcare team clear information about your problem and how you're progressing toward the ultimate goal: pickleball mastery! Well, at least the ability to play friendly club games without your elbow feeling like it's getting roasted by an acetylene torch.

Performance Longevity Dashboard indicators should help predict outcomes.

An easy way to summarize this precept is "if this, then that." As you better understand the indicator lights that are lighting up on your body's dashboard, you can more directly connect your behaviors and experiences with their outcomes. Identifying these relationships more clearly can turn lagging indicators like chronic pain into leading indicators like quantifiable changes in range of motion. Let's return for a moment to your pickleball-itis situation.

After a thorough exam, the doctor says you've got lateral epicondylitis (aka tennis elbow—or, in this case, pickleball elbow) and sends you off to physical therapy. Your PT uses all manner of therapeutic techniques: ultrasound, muscle scraping, and stretching and strengthening exercises. They also inform you that this particular variety of elbow annoyance is often caused by bad backhand form. How dare they?! Your backhand is perfect! Except you can't seem to get the ball to go where you want it to go when you return serves—but it's definitely not because you swing your arm and guess.

As it turns out, an arm-heavy backhand that doesn't properly align the torso is a pretty good predictor for tennis (pickleball) elbow. If you remember from Chapter 1, form is a leading indicator. Having a lackluster backhand doesn't mean you *will* get pickleball elbow, just that you're *more likely* to get it. So, if you want to avoid flare-ups, then it might be worth your while to clean up that stroke. Furthermore, when you notice your form beginning to break down on your ninety-ninth match of the week, you'll know *if* you don't change your course of action, *then* your elbow is more likely to start hurting again. In other words, you're #trending (review page 41) toward elbow dysfunction. This may or may not result in you playing less pickleball, but you will have better information with which to either mitigate potential downsides of continuing to play stupidly or do something else. Leading indicators predict outcomes and keep you in the driver's seat so that when things happen, you don't think that they randomly landed on you like a freshly hatched ladybug.

Performance Longevity Dashboard indicators should determine impact.

Impact is a measurement of what matters. After eight weeks of physical therapy and some lessons with your local pickleball pro, you're feeling great. You no longer have elbow pain, and your slicing backhand is the talk of the town. Success is yours. Now it's on you to monitor your backhand skills so you don't slide back into your old, nefarious habits.

Conversely, if you go to physical therapy and do the exercises and then spend some time with a pickleball pro who tunes up your backhand and you *still* have pain when you play (and can't manage to get the damn ball to go where you want), then it's time to reevaluate the plan. These lagging indicators let you know if you are achieving your goals and measuring up to the standard you set out. All of the fancy therapeutic interventions in the world don't mean much if they're not having a measurable effect on the outcomes you care about most.

When creating a Personal Longevity Dashboard, it can be difficult to decide where to start and what's important. It can be helpful to have a simple model that buckets your physiological experience into bite-sized pieces. Taking on every marker, indicator, and measure and trying to fit it all into a dashboard is way too much to manage even for those with sophisticated knowledge and education. Creating simple organizational categories will help anchor you in a practice that you can use in real life rather than get stuck in the mire of nerdgineering. To do this, we're going to use the M3 Model.

ORGANIZING INDICATORS: THE M3 MODEL

The purpose of the M3 Model is to help you organize the innumerable signals from your body that you have to contend with at any given time into digestible categories. The M3 Model has three categories: MIND, MoVeMenT, and MaTTeR. Think of these categories as buckets from which you can pull indicators to place on your dashboard.

- MIND is the collection of our internal thoughts, feelings, and perceptions. For the purposes of this book, we're going to avoid the esoteric, mystical, and unmeasurable and instead stick to the layers of our neurobiology and how they collaborate to produce our thinking and behavior—especially with regard to how we are affected by and adapt to stress. While this layer is often the most difficult to contend with, even small improvements in awareness ripple through our entire experience as humans. The effects of our thoughts, feelings, and perceptions on our performance longevity cannot be overstated.

- MVMT is the navigation of your body in space and time. It's how we orient our juicy meat suit through the environment to solve problems as well as express ourselves emotionally and aesthetically. Many of us don't pay much attention to our bodies until something below the surface shoots off a flare in the form of pain, dysfunction, or system failure that finally gets us to take notice. If you develop indicators that work in daily life as part of an integrative health practice, you can get ahead of trouble.

- MTTR refers to your biochemistry—your molecular health as measured through biomarkers found in blood work. There is an incredible orchestration of self-organizing chemistry happening inside the human body every second. It's so effective that there's energy left over for the organism (that's you) to read this book, make sense of it, and choose whether or not to change your behavior. There's much talk in popular health culture about markers for longevity. What should we pay attention to? How should we keep track of it all and act on it while we get on with life? More on that yet to come.

Although I've prescribed specific names and attributes to each category of the M3 Model, it's essential to remember that in reality, the three categories are interwoven into one human being. I only emphasize each of them separately for the sake of easier understanding, communication, and effectiveness. In truth, if the needle moves on one, there are simultaneous reverberations that echo throughout the entire person.

Throughout this book, I'll use these categories as buckets to collect different indicators, and I hope you'll keep using these buckets long after you're done with this book to help organize your health and performance with greater ease. As you do, please keep in mind that the most important thing is the synergy that occurs when aspects of each are managed as part of a whole.

In the coming chapters, you'll use the M3 Model to build the specifics of your dashboard. We'll go into each category to spend time unpacking the concepts along with case studies and anecdotes. As we do so, we'll continue to reinforce the three original precepts: bring clarity to problems, predict outcomes, and determine impact.

Simply being aware of what's going on under the hood isn't enough, though, is it? It's great to know why you're pulled over on the side of the road, but knowing that your timing belt is busted doesn't exactly complete the circle in this situation. Not only do you need a dashboard of indicators to improve your awareness, but you also need tools that help you maintain this vehicle and address problems if and when they arise. For each set of indicators in the M3 Model, it's helpful to have some tools on tap to fix the issue or, at minimum, to abashedly roll the vehicle into the mechanic's parking lot.

With that in mind, you don't have to know all of the indicators and have all of the tools (seeing as how that's impossible and all). What does help is having a good mechanic or two that you trust in your corner. That said, having some basic knowledge about what indicator lights are going off and what tools you've already tried to fix the problem will help you have more informed conversations with specialists if and when the need arises.

Onward, upward, forward.

SELF-REFLECTION QUESTIONS

In the arena of health and performance, what are some things you can identify as problems you might want to solve or goals you might want to achieve? Describe them as clearly and precisely as you can.

_____

_____

How can the outcome(s) you're striving for be measured? In other words, what KPIs can be attached to them?

_____

_____

How could tracking this KPI(s) be used to predict outcomes?

_____

_____

How could tracking this KPI(s) be used to determine impact?

_____

_____

What signals—in the form of KPIs—are on your current dashboard?

_____

_____

What do those signals do?

_____

_____

Are any warning signals flashing?

_____

_____

What KPIs on your dashboard are the most measurable? What is the unit of measurement?

_____

_____

What do the KPIs tell you about how your body is working now? What information do they provide about what might happen in the future?

_____

_____

Think carefully about why you rely on those indicators. What makes them reliable? Where might they be limited?

_____

_____

> **"**We become what we behold. We shape
> our tools and then our tools shape us."
> —**Marshall McLuhan**

CHAPTER 3: | Tools

Let's take a moment to revisit the story from the beginning of the book. You're driving along, everything is hunky-dory, and then—bam!— you're on the side of the road. You get out to see what's amiss and find that you have a flat tire. The tire pressure sensor has been illuminated for weeks, but I won't beat you up about that right now. When you see that flat tire, you think, *I got my Honor Scout merit badge in basic auto maintenance. I can fix this.*

You remember the steps to change a tire as clear as day. You need to loosen the lug nuts, jack the car up to get the tire off the ground, take the lug nuts off, replace the tire, start the lug nuts, drop the tire back down, and then tighten the lug nuts the rest of the way. You know what the problem is, and you know the solution, but in order to implement that solution, you need something else: tools. A simple lug wrench and jack are included with every motor vehicle. Why? They are the necessary tools for the most basic problem drivers are likely to encounter, and they're easy to use. Some of us may have a few more tools in an on-board toolkit—wrenches, screwdrivers, mallets, etc.—probably based on our knowledge and experience of repairing motor vehicles (and whether or not our auto insurance policy includes roadside assistance).

The point is, it's not enough to know your indicators, whether they arrive early enough for you to course-correct or not. You also need a toolkit so you can handle the basic maintenance and repair required for your own performance longevity. Whether it is prayer and meditation for the mind, stretches to keep pain and stiffness at bay, or a reliable way to improve your nutrition, upkeep and repair of your body and mind is your responsibility, just like it is with your car. A basic toolkit gives you the resources you need to keep the system in tip-top shape and address simple problems if and when they arise. It can be easy, however, to get caught up in the whirlwind of chasing gadgets to solve problems without giving enough due consideration to what tools should be in your toolbox in the first place.

THE THREE Rs OF TOOL SELECTION

Just as you use the M3 Model to organize your indicators, you use the three Rs to choose the best tools for your toolkit. The three Rs are

- Robust

- Reliable

- Repeatable

I first heard these terms from my friend Mickey Schuch. Mick is one of the best teachers of anything I've ever seen. Through his company, Carry Trainer, Mick teaches civilians everything from proper and lawful firearms use for personal protection to emergency medical skills. He helps prepare his students for the worst days they may ever face, and he does it very well. I've heard stories from returning students who left training events and used the skills they learned from Mick to save lives.

One of the things I like most about how Mick teaches is that it's not just a bunch of shoot-'em-up, cool guy, macho nonsense. There's a thoughtful philosophy behind everything he does, and the selection of tools and skills he chooses to use and teach are no exception. That's where the three Rs come in. In Mick's classes, when we talk about what tools we might want to carry with us, which skills we should invest time in learning, or what systems we use to deploy those tools, the criteria are, "Are they robust? Are they reliable? Are they repeatable?"

The more I pondered it, the more I realized that these criteria are applicable to any kind of toolkit. In fact, if you've used tools in a specific domain like automotive repair, law enforcement, or the military, chances are you will automatically run things through this filter over time. What we often fail to do is apply this filter to tools outside our area of expertise, and it makes us less efficient—or, worse, sometimes we lose faith in our ability to fix problems altogether.

Let's examine each of the Rs in a bit more detail. To help bring as much clarity to these ideas as possible, I am going to lean on the worlds of engineering and scientific research.

Robust

In engineering terms, robustness is "the ability of a system to withstand external demands or perturbations without degradation in functionality." Robust materials are harder to break and can withstand hard use and even abuse. We've all bought and used tools that weren't made to stand the test of time—that kitchen knife that won't hold an edge or the trash bags with drawstrings that rip out (I hate that). Conversely, we revere tools that "take a lickin' and keep on tickin'" like the Timex watch, the Toyota Land Cruiser (beloved by warlords across continents), and the ubiquitous Swiss Army Knife. The value of such tools is their ability to last through the worst of it. It's for this reason that I've recommended lacrosse balls to special operators and athletes for well over a decade in spite of advancements in self-massage tools. For the most part, they get the job done, and they are impossible to break (and even really difficult to drill through—I've tried).

In addition to the physical makeup of a tool, robustness can refer to systems, strategies, and solutions. Does the way that a plan or system is being implemented stand up to potential interference? For example, robustness in manufacturing means that a chain of procedures leading to the production of a certain quantity and quality of a product by a certain date will in fact deliver said products as described in spite of potential breakdown in the manufacturing chain. The more robust the process, the more things can go wrong before the entire system breaks down, and the easier it is to get things back online should they fail.

This same concept of robustness can be helpful when it comes to deciding what kinds of tools you're going to use in the pursuit of performance longevity. For example, will your new $2,000 massage chair withstand your four-dog household? If not, you'd better find a different way to deal with the restless leg syndrome that keeps you up nights. Additionally, the system you have in place to deal with the buzzing jumpiness in your sore legs should be one that you can easily adapt to as many circumstances as you find yourself in. If your plan can only be executed in a specific way, with a specific item, at a specific time and place, your plan is not robust and often will not be executed with enough consistency to make a dent in your goals.

This may seem like overkill, but many times in the course of my career I have seen people latch on to fragile strategies for health and performance, and when those strategies fail, the entire house of cards comes tumbling down. Complete reliance on apps, supplements, fancy gadgetry, or specific environmental conditions is a recipe for failure in the long term.

As a personal anecdote, I do my best to keep my sleep hygiene routine when I'm on the road teaching seminars as similar as possible to when I'm at home. Within a sixty- to ninety-minute window prior to closing my eyes, I gradually downshift my activity, dim the lights in the house, and do some foam rolling or stretching. This strategy works quite well for me personally, not to mention that it is robust enough that small changes in the rest of my day don't flush this process down the toilet whether I'm going to sleep in my own bed that night or in a hotel bed in some distant land.

Robustness is strength, sturdiness, and stability. Robust things are hard to break. They are the opposite of fragile. Robust can describe what the tool itself is made of but also refers to systems, processes, and solutions that can withstand and overcome adversity. Not every tool you use has to be in the Robustness Hall of Fame, but it's definitely a quality worth considering.

Reliable

Leaning on engineering once again, reliability is "the probability that a product or system will perform its intended function adequately for a given period of time." In other words, reliable means you can expect consistent and predictable results over time. If a tool is reliable, it will perform under specific conditions with little to no failure. While reliability might seem to overlap with robustness, they are a bit different. Robustness refers to durability, and reliability refers to a consistent outcome. A reliable friend has been there when you need them over and over again. They deliver on their promises. Reliable tools are the same.

Toyota automobiles are well known for their dependability (aka reliability). In February 2024, J.D. Power released its annual U.S. Vehicle Dependability Study (VDS). The primary scoring system of the VDS is known as the pp100, or problems per 100 vehicles. While on average all automotive manufacturers' pp100 scores have worsened due to the increase in complex computer and infotainment technology, one company stands head and shoulders above the rest: Toyota. The Japanese automaker scored a 135 with its luxury brand, Lexus, and a 147 for its name-brand automobiles. Buick was a close second with 149, and everybody else ranked far behind. This is why, year after year, Toyotas dominate American highways—because if you own one and you turn the key or push the start button, the engine hums without fail. That's reliability.

I want to step back to emphasize a key phrase in the original engineering definition: "intended function." This phrase speaks to the first rule of the Performance Longevity Dashboard: "Bring clarity to problems and identify outcomes." Too often when people decide to use a tool for pain relief, engage in an exercise, or digest a supplement, they skip over the "intended function" part. Before you can possibly know if anything is delivering a consistent result for you, you must know the result you are looking for and how you are going to measure it. If you're not sure, get help. And don't be afraid to try. Just be sure to try with a why.

Let's bring this back around to how you might consider reliability when it comes to the tools you might use to stay healthy and perform better.

First, you have to identify what it is that you are after. Maybe you want to sleep better—specifically, you want to improve deep sleep. You decide to use your Apple Watch to track your sleep for the next two weeks. You start taking GABA, a neurotransmitter that reduces excitability in mammalian nervous systems and can be taken as a supplement before bed. After a few days, you notice that your sleep has measurably improved, and you feel more well rested and less sore in the morning. You don't take GABA all the time, but over the next six months, you use it intermittently in different contexts and find that when you do take it, you get the same results. You now have a reliable tool that helps improve your sleep. In the workbook at the back of this book, you are going to have a chance to try personal health experiments like the one I just described and learn how to construct your own experiments, too.

When picking tools to remedy health issues and boost performance, reliability is an important consideration. On its face, this statement probably seems obvious, and on a page in a book it is. But many times in my career, I have watched clients use tools that deliver mixed results because an online talking head recommended it or because their friend uses it or because it's just what they thought they were supposed to do. Be sure that you know what it is you're shooting for and how you are going to measure it, and then pay attention to whether or not the tool you picked for the job is a reliable one. Be sure you know how to use those tools properly too—which brings us to the last of the three Rs.

Repeatable

In science and engineering, repeatability is a measure of the likelihood that, having produced one result from an experiment, you can try the same experiment, with the same setup, and produce that exact same result. Reliability is often interchanged with the term *reproducibility*, which is "a measure of whether results in a [research] paper can be attained by a different research team, using the same methods." This shows that the results obtained are not artifacts of the unique setup in one research lab but rather that the procedure being used for the experiment can be repeated with accuracy.

If we apply this idea to the deployment of tools that will help performance longevity, it means the procedure with which we deploy those tools needs to be standardized and therefore repeatable. In short, do you know the order of operations for the use of the tool in question? A simple example is in the methods you might use to improve your range of motion through stretching.

I've spent a good portion of my career as a manual therapist and a strength and conditioning coach helping athletes alleviate basic movement and pain problems. One technique we used quite often was PNF stretching. (PNF is short for proprioceptive neuromuscular facilitation. Yeah, PNF is easier.) PNF uses the nerve tissues inside the bellies and tendons of muscles to facilitate a sort of soft reset of those tissues to improve range of motion. It's well researched, widely accepted, and, best of all, easy to learn and use. PNF gets very predictable positive outcomes (ahem—reliability), but you have to do the steps correctly.

The steps are as follows:

1. Control your breathing.
2. Take the tissues you want to improve to their pain-free end range of motion.
3. Take a deep inhale and hold it.
4. Create a contraction in the tissues.
5. Exhale slowly and with control.
6. Take the tissues to the newly available pain-free end range of motion and hold.
7. Repeat steps 1–6 to satisfactory change.

This process is easy to deploy, especially after you've practiced it a few times, and it can be used darn near anywhere you're feeling stiff without negative repercussions. However, you have to do it with focus and intention in the given order or your results will be severely limited. I've heard many athletes try to make the case that it didn't work for them only to find out they were skipping steps or giving insufficient attention to the process. I don't mean to say that PNF is some sort of panacea that will heal all that ails you if you do it right. What I am saying is that you cannot expect any tool, process, or intervention to perform with optimal reliability if you do not execute the use of that tool with care. With that in mind, it's essential to ask yourself a couple of key questions when you begin to apply a new tool, especially one that has implications for the functionality of the body you live in:

- Do I know what I'm trying to change and how to measure it?

- Can I adequately repeat the steps of this process to achieve consistent outcomes?

Over the course of my career, one bottleneck has come up over and over again with nearly all health and performance interventions: user implementation. The best medicine, supplement, or gadget means nothing if the user doesn't know how and when to apply it for optimal results. Furthermore, you have to be willing to take responsibility for the skilled application of any intervention you choose. Health and performance longevity are not hands-off-the-wheel ventures.

PROXIMAL TO DISTAL

Overlapping the three Rs for tool selection is the concept of proximal and distal tools. Proximal tools are the ones that are going to be the most accessible, the most often. This means you can use them with lots of frequency if and when you need to. Distal tools are on the periphery of your toolkit. They are things you have access to less often and so shouldn't rely on as primary ways to solve problems. Imagine the concentric rings of an archery target with you standing right on the bullseye. The tools closest to you in the center are your proximal tools. Those are the tools that you'll invest the most time and energy in and rely on the most.

Proximal tools are kept at arm's reach so that you can use them to take care of yourself. My proximal tools are the foam roller by my bed and the kettlebell in my kitchen. Foam rollers don't by any means solve all orthopedic pain problems, but mine lets me get some quality work in on my soft tissues before I go to sleep. By the same token, the kettlebell that lives next to my cutlery isn't the only way I challenge my body to get stronger, but I know that no matter what else happens, I can count on it to be there every day if I want to get some quality strength training done.

Distal tools are not as readily available, so your reliance on them should be minimal for the most part. Distal tools aren't necessarily less effective than proximal tools. They are often more specialized in nature and are made to solve specific types of problems, or they are more complicated in their use or harder to access. I'm fortunate enough to do most of my exercise training at Virginia High Performance in Virginia Beach. At VHP, they have all manner of awesome, high-tech exercise equipment like vibration plates for specific nervous system stimulation and cable resistance machines that offer fixed-load resistance to minimize momentum and enhance proprioception. They're pretty cool when I'm there, nobody else is using them, and I remember how to use them properly. Great tools, but not centerpieces in my approach to staying healthy.

Misplacing tools on the continuum of proximal to distal can leave us vulnerable to over-reliance on external solutions. I'll give you an example from my experience. People I worked with in clinical settings would say things to me like, "Oh, I used to go to a massage therapist to get my back worked on every week, but ever since so-and-so went on maternity leave, I've really gone downhill." Tools like this can be taken away without warning, leaving you more vulnerable to potential downturns in functionality. The best massage therapist in the world cannot help you if they aren't at work. Distal tools, even when they are effective on their own, may not add to the robustness of your performance longevity system if you rely on them too much. The tools that are most proximal to you should be the ones that are the most robust, reliable, and repeatable.

Another upside of applying this concept is that it keeps the locus of control close to you. That means you maintain a course of action that you know is reliable—literally and figuratively within arm's reach. This might seem like a bit of analytical overkill when it comes to something as seemingly benign as which tools you will put in your performance longevity toolkit, but I can assure you that it is not. Many times I have seen people regress in pain, weight management, fitness, and performance because they relied on distal tools as anchors for their health.

When I worked as a sports massage therapist some years ago, I had a couple of clients who were professional soccer players. As you might imagine, these athletes were incredibly talented and had regular access to trainers, coaches, and physical therapists over the course of their time playing. A downside of all this access was that they had no strategies for self-care and were nearly helpless without external intervention. This culminated in a call to me on a Sunday afternoon when one of these athletes reported that she needed "an emergency massage," to which I responded that there is no such thing. Emergencies are for doctors, nurses, and first responders. In this case, this athlete had no proximal strategies for addressing her own basic recovery needs, which made her vulnerable when situations arose and external help was unavailable. More proximal strategies like foam rolling, stretching, and sauna would have been more appropriate under those conditions. Again, it's not that it is wrong to have effective and specialized distal tools. It's just less effective to rely on tools that are not as accessible as go-to solutions.

My point in explaining this idea of proximal to distal isn't to tell you which tools to put where. That's ultimately for you to decide. It is a simple framework to help you determine which tools you will include in your toolbox and how much time, energy, and trust you will invest in each of them. Examples of proximal tools can vary by context, individual needs and preferences, and skill. For me, a chainsaw is a distal tool that I keep in my shed and rarely use in my suburban life. It's on an outer ring of that target for sure. But if you're a lumberjack, a chainsaw is right in the center of that ring for you. Similarly, a professional athlete may have free and regular access to a float tank to help them get into a state of deep relaxation whenever they need it, whereas the rest of us might need to pay out of pocket and take time out of our busy family and work lives to access such a tank and with a lot less frequency—in which case we would need another way to access states of deep relaxation for our own benefit.

Remember, too, that your proximal and distal tools may change over time. Just like any other tools you keep around, trial and error will inform which tools you use for health and performance longevity and under what conditions. What's important to know is that you should invest the vast majority of your time, energy, and trust in the tools you are going to rely on with the most frequency under the most conditions.

While these concepts are covered explicitly here, the goal is that over time, they become implicit parts of your thinking when you're deciding whether or not a device or method will become a part of the toolkit that you use to keep yourself performing your best. Keep asking yourself these questions:

- Is this tool robust?

- Is it reliable?

- Is it repeatable?

- Under what conditions will I have access to it?

The concepts outlined in this chapter can be quite intuitive when practiced diligently. Often, when we are taught how to use tools for our job or as part of a hobby, they are implicit in the instruction we receive. For example, if you're a firefighter, you receive clear instruction on how to use the tools you are issued as part of that job. Unfortunately, it is not common practice to get equipped with the tools you need to support performance longevity. The purpose of stating them clearly and explicitly here is to ensure that you use these ideas to engage with the most important thing you'll ever take care of—your own health.

In the coming chapters, we are going to dig deep into the M3 Model as well as look at examples of tools that can help you maintain various aspects of your performance longevity. As you read, keep these ideas in mind. I encourage you to come back to this chapter from time to time as a way to keep the basics cemented in your thinking.

SELF-REFLECTION QUESTIONS

Name some examples of tools that you use, whether for work or at home, that are robust, reliable, and repeatable. How do you know that those tools fit each of those criteria?

_____

_____

List some tools that you use in your daily life and note which ones are proximal and which are distal. Why does each tool fit into that category?

_____

_____

Are there tools that you already use to support your performance longevity that fit into these categories? What are they? Take a few minutes to write three or four sentences about them.

_____

_____

_____

_____

SECTION TWO
THE M3 MODEL

Before you dig into Section Two, which goes into depth on each of the three gauges on the dashboard and the indicators that are used, I'd like to provide some guidance on how to get the most out of this information. There are two main ways to go about navigating Section Two and its three chapters, each devoted to one of the Ms in the M3 Model:

- You can read straight through as you normally would read a book and save any further investigation for after completion.

- You can work through each chapter while filling out the corresponding section of the workbook at the same time, devote some thought and study to how each of the topics applies to you, and then move on to the next M in the M3 Model.

Neither approach is necessarily better than the other, but I will emphasize that using the workbook to take notes and answer key questions while you read through the chapters in this section will help you discover which indicators work best for you and determine how to go about deploying them to improve your health and performance.

Which brings me to my next point: Please don't take the examples and case studies as gospel. They're included simply to illustrate the points at hand and provide a reference for indicators backed by sound research and experience. The real trick is to use the underlying lessons to develop your own dashboard over time, even if you start with the ones I talk about in this book. There are literally too many potential indicators—even good ones—to list, so continue to learn, explore, and adapt well beyond this book.

Lastly, don't hesitate to seek out additional information from trusted sources. The same way you'd consult a mechanic you trust to get more information about what's going on with your car when you want to know how to do a better job of maintaining and repairing it, I encourage you to build a network of subject matter experts and advisors with whom you can discuss the indicators on your dashboard and what to do about them when they come on.

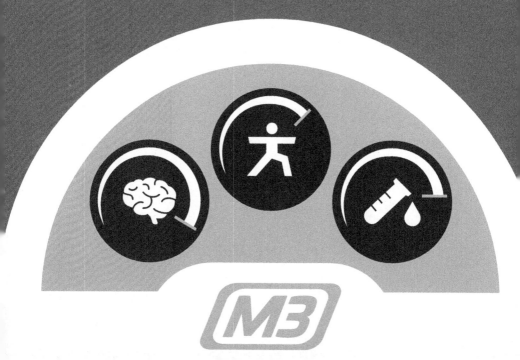

> **"** *Your vision will become clear only when you look into your own heart. Who looks outside, dreams; who looks inside, awakes.*"
>
> —C. G. Jung

CHAPTER 4: | MIND

The human mind is elusive even under the modern microscope of neuroscience, psychology, and philosophy. After all, your mind is studying itself. This fact can make it extremely difficult to manage the thoughts, feelings, and behaviors that drive so much of internal human experience. As complex as it is, nobody can deny the power and influence of the mind when it comes to sustaining performance and health for a lifetime.

Not too long ago, I asked my friend and legendary track and field coach Dan Pfaff what he believes is the greatest limiter of performance on game day. His answer: emotional challenges, especially those intertwined with family or relationship stress. That's right, it wasn't nutritional imperfection, faulty training sessions, or even injury. It was emotional disruption brought on by relationships.

If you've ever had your life thrown into disarray by familial or relationship issues, this answer probably doesn't come as a big surprise, but in an ironic twist, we seldom take proactive steps to attend to our own psycho-emotional well-being. It doesn't have to be like that, though. You don't have to settle for the kind of drag in your performance that a lack of care in the realm of MIND will surely create. There are indicators you can put on your Performance Longevity Dashboard that will give you valid, reliable, and accessible information about what's going on in your brain and mind that lead you to actionable steps for improving yourself.

The topic of the human mind is a vast area of study. For centuries, priests, philosophers, poets, psychologists, and scientists have pondered what the mind is and how it works. Right out of the gate, I want to be clear about something: my intention with this chapter is not to encapsulate anything even remotely representing a complete view of the mind. Instead, we'll explore a framework that provides an opportunity to develop knowledge, skills, and practices that tangibly and measurably improve health, life, and performance for the long haul.

With that in mind (pun intended), I'll use the layers of the nervous system and their commensurate functions as the anchor point for this exploration. The use of these layers serves multiple purposes:

- First, if you have a better understanding of what the layers are, you can become more aware of their effects on you.

- Second, each layer offers an opportunity to create a key performance indicator. If you can measure it, you can change it.

- Lastly, each layer has an explicit and important relationship to how you process stress—which brings me to my next point regarding MIND in the context of performance longevity.

In my experience, poor relationships with stress are some of the most limiting factors in all of health and performance, and there's plenty of data to back me up. It probably comes as no surprise that stress and anxiety are at an all-time cultural high. Is it because the world is such a mess or because our ancient physiology is unfamiliar with the demands placed on us by the rapid technological advancements that we are experiencing? Or is it that modern life is too easy and "this generation is soft"?

Regardless of the origin, about which there are as nearly as many opinions as actual contributing factors, one reality remains: we all experience stress. Having a better understanding of the factors involved in your subconscious processing systems and how you can become more aware of those so you can alter how you think, feel, and act for the better is what this chapter is all about. I'll cover some indicators that are known to be helpful

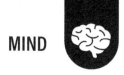

additions to the Performance Longevity Dashboard as well as some sensible and accessible tools that are backed by best practice and good science.

THE TRIUNE BRAIN

In an effort to make this vast topic more digestible, I am going to lean on the Triune Brain model from neuroscientist Paul MacClean. This model, originally proposed by Dr. MacClean in 1964, offers an explanation of the human brain according to three layers of evolutionary timeline and function. From most ancient to most recent, Dr. MacClean labeled them the Reptilian (basal ganglia), Paleomammalian (limbic), and Neomammalian (cortical) brains. Each layer has its own distinct set of functions and constituent structures as determined by the necessity of evolution. While I won't use this exact model for this category of indicators, it served as an inspiration for my thinking as I wrote this chapter.

Full disclosure: The Triune Brain model has long been known to be an inaccurate representation of neuroanatomical reality based on up-to-date evidence. When viewed through the lens of neuroscience, that's true. The various functions of the nervous system and brain co-evolved with intertwining form and structure. The Triune Brain is woefully incomplete from a purely technical standpoint. With that said, it does provide a latticework that can be helpful for constructing a working model of the brain and nervous system, especially in regard to becoming a more conscious architect of both your inner life and your outward behavior. A map is not a precise representation of land, but that does not render it useless. Having a working model that points toward usable heuristics can be helpful to encourage a journey toward awareness and exploration. To that end, I'll use the Triune Brain as a point of departure for this discussion.

The Three Layers of MIND

Like Dr. MacClean's Triune Brain, I'll define MIND in terms of three interconnected layers: the autonomic, the emotional, and the cognitive. Each layer represents a set of distinct but overlapping modi operandi. As we move forward, we'll take a deeper look at each layer and how the layers interact, especially in terms of how they influence your relationship with performance longevity. Additionally, I'll talk about some specific indicators for each layer and how you may be able to integrate those into your Performance Longevity Dashboard.

A key point should remain in the backdrop as this chapter temporarily isolates each tier of MIND. In no reality do these operational systems exist as islands unto themselves. The three layers are braided together in the beautifully orchestrated expression of what it means to be a thinking, feeling human being. These layers interact both functionally and structurally to create the pantheon of feeling and behavior that we exhibit in real life. I make this point for this reason: Singular, direct answers are easier to deal with than complex ones. When we key in on a particular aspect of MIND, we can tend to isolate a specific anatomical area or function and attribute its malfunction as the cause of our distress or its development as the source of our success. Doing so neglects the big picture and can leave us open to blind spots on our road to performance longevity. Zoom in for understanding, zoom out for application.

The Autonomic Layer

The autonomic nervous system (ANS) is the most fundamental layer of our neurobiology. *Autonomic* is derived from the word *autonomy*, which refers to self-governance. For all intents and purposes, your ANS can and does operate without conscious influence from you. It drives fundamental physiological processes that keep you alive, such as heart rate, breathing, blood flow, and digestion. These core behaviors manage the necessary chemistry of life on autopilot through feedback loops that are built into

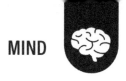

your body from birth and then shaped further by behavioral inputs that you accrue over a lifetime.

The ANS functions on a simple and straightforward biological directive: survive and replicate. This edict is at the center of all animal behavior. From this, a nearly infinite variety of expressions may emerge depending on the attributes of the particular organism and the way in which it interacts with its environment. This biological reality is an essential concept to consider as we begin to contextualize both the way humans operate in general and the subtle costs that stress load can take on our physiology, often without our conscious awareness. That is, until the engine starts smoking...

The malfunctioning of this core physiology contributes to numerous problems and is caused not only by the quality of the foods you eat and the rest you get, but also by the way you deal with the stress of life. Managing stress effectively can mean the difference between remaining resilient and adaptable and breaking down toward disease and discontent.

> *"'How did you go bankrupt?' 'Two ways. Gradually and then suddenly.'"*
>
> **—Ernest Hemingway,** *The Sun Also Rises*

The autonomic nervous system is further subdivided into two complementary anatomical and functional groups: the sympathetic nervous system and the parasympathetic nervous system. These two subsystems offer both unique anatomical components as well as differing functional aspects. For the purposes of this book, I'm not going to go too deep into the anatomy, as the language around it can become esoteric and steer us away from our core purpose. There are volumes of books directed at this endeavor, and if you want to become an expert driver, I encourage you to check out the Resources section for more information. Having a basic understanding of the sympathetic and parasympathetic, however, can help you navigate your mind more effectively when it comes to how you interact with and adapt to stress, especially under the conditions of this modern environment.

Gas and Brakes: Driving the Autonomic Nervous System

Let's begin with the sympathetic nervous system (SNS). The sympathetic is governed by the four Fs. Fight and flight are the two that get the most press, but they don't run the entire show. Alongside them are freeze and fornicate. (Freeze is sympathetic because even though the outside is still, the internal physiology is going a hundred miles per hour. Think of your heart racing while you hide behind a bush from a grizzly bear.) The SNS activates your physiology. It's about using energy for action. The sympathetic makes things like heart rate, breathing, and blood pressure increase. An easy way to think of the SNS is that it's like the gas pedal of your body.

The parasympathetic nervous system (PSNS) is the other half of the equation. The PSNS is the home of rest, digest, and recover. When the parasympathetic is the dominating force, you are in a state of conservation, repair, and rebuilding. If the SNS is activation, the PSNS is deactivation. The parasympathetic affects all of the same physiology as the sympathetic, but in the opposite direction. Things like heart rate, breathing, and blood pressure all decrease in a state of parasympathetic dominance. If the sympathetic is the gas pedal, the parasympathetic is the brake.

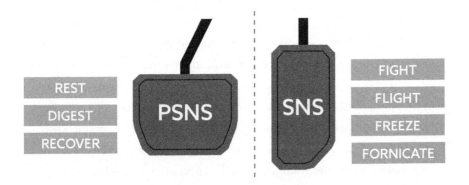

Most of the time, when we talk about these two components of our physiology, we think of them in terms of extremes. The sympathetic is the zebra running from the hungry lion on the savanna (flight). The parasympathetic is the yogi meditating in a monastery (rest). While these examples are technically correct, they represent static images that can be misleading and, to be blunt, disempowering. Rather than a pair of singular end states, it is far more helpful to think about the autonomic nervous system as a continuum. As you are reading this book right now, you are more sympathetic than when you first woke up this morning (pre-caffeination is assumed) but less sympathetic than you would be when sprinting to your departure gate so you don't miss your flight.

Just like driving is more nuanced than simply putting the pedal to the metal or slamming on the brakes, so too is your autonomic physiology. You glide back and forth along the continuum of neurological arousal in the same way that you accelerate smoothly when the light turns green and coast to a stop when it's red. While the autonomic nervous system does function on its own, it is possible to become skilled at directing it through conscious behaviors that you adopt. Then, just like getting better at driving, you can more effectively decide whether you want gas or brakes, how much you want, and when. The ability to move back and forth is important for a healthy and balanced autonomic nervous system and is the foundation of how your body adapts to the stressors that life brings.

It's not the proverbial saber-toothed tiger crouching in the Paleolithic megaflora that makes people hit this gas these days. More and more, it is the compounding and insidious modern stimuli that keep the gas pedal down longer than it needs to be, burning up more fuel than you would otherwise require. Artificial light, chronically disrupted sleep, constant stimulation from electronic devices, copious consumption of stimulants—the list goes on. It's not that a state of sympathetic activation is inherently bad, just as having a car that can go fast is not inherently bad; it's that gunning the engine uses more energy and is expensive.

The SNS evolved for bursts of activation that drive you into action. It's the thing that mobilizes your body to sprint toward the sound when you hear your child start screaming in the backyard. When misappropriated, though, it wears heavily on those same physiological systems that it powers. It is well documented that when chronically activated, the SNS contributes to gastrointestinal problems, cardiovascular disease, and anxiety, among other unwanted health issues. You absolutely need sympathetic drive, but in order to drive with skill, you need brakes, too. Which brings us back to the parasympathetic nervous system.

The PSNS gets a lot of press these days. There are wearable devices and smartphone apps that tell you how well rested you are and when you need a break. More and more businesses are even providing days off for mental health and support for dealing with stress. For the most part, I think this is a good thing. Life in the information age is a far cry from our ancestral environment, with less natural opportunity for rest and repose. As a result, it's important to develop keen sensitivities and robust skills for moving the needle toward rest and recovery when you need to.

The most obvious example of a parasympathetic state is sleep (assuming it is healthy and restorative). Brain and body focus energy expenditure inward to rebuild the hardware and reboot the software. The ability to modulate your internal state is a skill that saves you massive amounts of energy over the long haul in order to better respond to stress, whether it's an emergency situation or a psychological burden brought on by the normal stuff of life.

Building on the Autonomic

Our ancient ancestors relied far more heavily on the autonomic simplicity of gas and brakes to regulate their environmental navigation. Over time, biological evolution gave rise to newer neurological systems like the limbic and cortical structures that allowed humans to develop more sophisticated approaches to solving the problems of living longer and perpetuating their genes. As we explore the next two layers of MIND, remember that regardless of how intelligent the systems get, they have deep functional as well as anatomical connections to their physiological predecessors.

Realizing this, you can more readily tune in to physiological indicators when they light up on your dashboard. Later in this chapter as well as in the workbook, we'll examine and experiment with some of those indicators. Integrating them into your dashboard can improve both your performance and your quality of life.

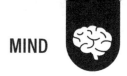

It's important to note that genetics, personal history, and personality type all play a role in which end of the autonomic spectrum you tend to operate on and what sorts of stimuli your gas and brake pedals tend to respond to as a result of those individual proclivities. As this chapter continues, we'll discuss cross-talk between the layers of MIND and how they work together to produce your experience of the world, especially with regard to how you deal with stress.

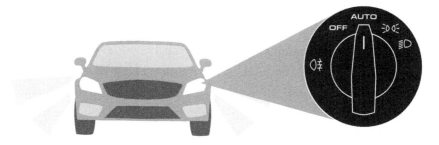

The Accountant: Stress Banking

When it comes to making this information useful and tying it into how you can better pay attention to and alter the effects that stress has on you, it's useful to know something very simple about your autonomic nervous system: It's an accountant. It doesn't care where your stress came from, just like an accountant doesn't really care about why you spent money, just that you did. How much did that cost? How much is in the bank? How much is coming in? When it comes to stress, the physiological "cost" is all the ANS cares about, too. It doesn't care about reasons, justifications, narratives, or contexts—only cost. Is cost all that truly matters in the final analysis? Of course not. That being said, having an idea of how much you're spending and how much money is coming in is going to help you maintain the budget and avoid going broke.

If you can connect to this deeper physiology and place reliable indicators of cost on your dashboard, you can make better decisions about how you spend your energy and attention. For example, many wearable devices, such as smartwatches and fitness trackers, measure heart rate variability

(HRV) and offer apps that help you observe your autonomic state over time. Toward the end of this chapter and in the workbook, we'll take a look at HRV as a reliable way to monitor autonomic nervous system behavior, specifically the relationship between the gas and brake pedals and what that number can tell you about how well you are handling stress.

The autonomic nervous system is a great place to start the discussion of MIND because it deals in hard physiology. That means it's fairly easy to measure and manipulate. Numerical values representing stress create real trends that you can follow, but by no means do they offer a complete picture of the human mind. Having at least equal importance is the major driver of your felt experience in life: your emotions. Human emotions are complex and at times difficult to articulate and even more difficult to manage. It can be helpful to understand what they are, where they come from, and how an increased awareness of them can help you achieve the things you want.

More Than a Feeling: The Emotional Layer

Like the autonomic nervous system, the emotional layer of MIND is a powerful influence on how you interact with the world as well your subjective internal experience of those interactions. That's what makes it so hard to study and even talk about emotions; you experience them in a personal way. The difficulty of measuring emotions has led to their marginalization in the hierarchy of importance in the hard sciences—that is, until very recently.

This low placement on the podium is ironic, because as much as we'd like to think humans are the most rational species on the planet, we are deeply influenced by our emotional states. Emotions like joy, rage, and sadness have the power to drastically alter the way you think and perceive your experiences. Brushing your teeth the night after you get a promotion at work feels very different from brushing your teeth the morning after your beloved dog dies. We all know this, yet few of us spend time and attention on teasing out habits of feeling, at least until the engine blows up in our faces.

Your fluid emotional states are driven by both internal and environmental signals that slide below the radar of your conscious mind, setting off programs of repetitive behavior that you can remain unaware of—sometimes over a lifetime and often to your detriment. Before you try to change how you feel, it helps to understand why you feel that way in the first place. Emotions are incredibly complex, and the most informed people in the world have come to a consensus on the topic: They're working on it. What is clear is that emotions are not evolutionary afterthoughts or some residue of psychological weakness that you need to learn to suppress in order to function at optimal levels. Not at all. More and more hard neuroscience research shows that emotional health and resilience are an essential part of quality of life and have a dramatic impact on things you value, like your ability to learn, engage in long-lasting and intimate relationships, and even maintain cognitive health as you age.

Often, emotions are experienced as a state of reaction. They sort of happen to you or in you as a result of an event or sometimes for what seems like no reason at all. That's all well and good if things are going your way, but it's easy to get stuck in cycles of feeling, thinking, and acting that don't serve you over the long haul. Consistent with the central theme of this book, developing better indicators for how you're feeling can help you become a more conscious participant in your own evolution. To get a better handle on this process, let's start with a working definition of emotions as well as a little biological history.

A Brief History of Feelings

If we accept the basic idea that emotions are a part of our evolutionary process, then we can trace their origin to other mammalian ancestors for biological survival purposes. Our emotional origins can be found in an area of the brain known as the rhinencephalon, or "nose brain." This part of the brain evolved in mammals to help modulate autonomic responses and generate internal sensations with regard to threats (is this place or thing dangerous?) and opportunities (is there food or a mate here?) and has deep structural and functional connections to sense of smell. Over the long timelines of biological evolution, the rhinencephalon morphed into what is now commonly referred to as the limbic system. This primarily includes the amygdala, the area of the brain known for modulating the fear response, and the hippocampus, an area essential to the formation of new memories. These two structures and other areas of the brain coordinate to create the vast and complex landscape of emotions modern humans experience every single day.

To Jaak Panksepp, the father of affective neuroscience, emotions at their most fundamental level represent internal feeling states and motivations that organize animal behavior in response to the environment. Fear, probably the most powerful emotion there is, helps you avoid bodily injury and death but can be extrapolated to truly scary things like public speaking. Furthermore, these affective states are measurable behaviors with neurological origins and are not simply an artifice of the mind that clever marketeers use to manipulate your buying habits. Some environmental challenges were so persistent that internal sensations emerged that served to more reliably direct behavior. Emotional valence moves us toward or away from stimuli (positive or negative valence, respectively). Interestingly, and a nod to the complex overlapping that I'll discuss more later, there are innate valences, like disgust relating to rotten food or dead animals, that can be altered by context, culture, and personal experience. Such is the story of emotions.

With that said, we have some innate drives that underlie our most complex motivations and feeling states. For example, Panksepp uses the term SEEKING to categorize emotions like desire, hope, and anticipation, which developed from the pursuit of food, water, warmth, sex, and social contact. This SEEKING system is just one component of the fundamental drivers of our feelings. If you want dive more deeply into this particular viewpoint, Panksepp's book *Affective Neuroscience* provides enlightening insight and makes a strong case for the scientific basis of emotional thought at its origins. It's not necessary to cover all of the ups, downs, and all-arounds of this science to engage in this discussion, however. What is important is to realize that the complex emotions you experience help you organize your behavior

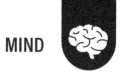

and solve problems. They're not a burden you must bear but instead are a necessary and, when harnessed, powerful asset to a more fulfilling existence and furthermore to expanding the resilience that allows you to actualize your potential.

Smell is a potent wizard

"Smell is a potent wizard that transports you across a thousand miles and all the years you have lived."

—Helen Keller

This quote beautifully summarizes an important aspect of emotion and its connection to our sense of smell. While we may not be driven as powerfully by smell as other mammals, there are powerful ties between our sense of smell, our emotions, and our memories. For me, the aroma of freshly baked bread teleports me immediately to my grandmother's kitchen. Not just the place and the memories, but all of the feelings of comfort and love a little boy getting a slice of fresh bread from his grandma feels. This connection between smell and emotions can trigger both positive and negative affectations. Not only that, but the ability to smell at all can have a direct effect on our cognitive capacity and emotional health. Anosmia, or loss of smell, was known to exacerbate symptoms for some people struggling with anxiety and depression during the COVID-19 pandemic, and bolstering the sense of smell is a promising route for treatment in improving memory and emotional regulation in some dementia patients.

It's Complex: Emotional Thinking, Ethics, Culture, and Learning

The storehouse of feelings that you use to navigate your world is largely a subconscious one that has deep roots in your personal history and is embedded within family and cultural environments. Emotional signals that originate very early in life can shape networks of behavior that in adulthood can be difficult to trace to their origins. It's hard to imagine a century-old oak tree as coming from a tiny acorn, but it does nonetheless. To that same end, a lightning strike or prevailing wind can alter the trajectory of that tree's growth, unbeknownst to the tree. During your earliest stages of life, much of the foundation of how you use your feelings is set. Genetics and environment intertwine to produce your internal map of the world and your basic idea of how you should interact with it. As with all of biology, both nature and nurture play a part. This is critical to understand because we often carry around our feelings and the amazing narratives that get wrapped around them without really understanding the purpose they serve for us.

Further layers of complexity reside in how we display our emotions and interact with others when they display theirs. For example, Japanese culture has a subdued external emotional delivery with volumes of subtext. Brazilians, by contrast, are boisterous and expressive by nature. These emotional tones have important effects on the lens through which various cultures view the world and make judgments about what constitutes appropriate feelings, thoughts, and behaviors. How you relate to yourself, your family, and your peers as well as your expectations of interacting with them color and reciprocally are colored by the culture you find yourself in. It's not that one kind is right and the other is wrong—that's certainly not the point. The point is that there are undercurrents of social emotion that affect the way you think, feel, and act. Furthermore, those things can and often do push and pull on your ability to perform well and stay healthy.

Not only does your social environment have an effect on you, but your need to be social does, too. Human beings are social animals and as a result have a strong innate need for kinship. The formation of bonds with your family and later your friends is an essential ingredient in your development as well as the long-term well-being that supports health and performance. While short-term loneliness due to social isolation has been shown to increase pro-social behavior and positive emotion when the lonely person reenters friend groups, long-term feelings of isolation perpetuate negative emotions and antisocial behavior. In his book *Tribe*, Sebastian Junger writes extensively on tribal anthropology and its connection to mental health disorders like PTSD for those who serve in uniform. This doesn't just hold true for those bonded in service, either. Prolonged feelings of isolation and disconnection are well known to exacerbate feelings of anxiety and depression in older adults, teens, and seemingly everybody in between. It seems that feeling lonely is fundamentally human.

Another point on the complexity of emotional life is how emotions affect learning. I don't necessarily mean your mood during pottery class here, but that certainly does play a role in your ability to take on new information. More specifically, I mean how meaning-making, relevance, and interest play crucial roles in what and how you learn. True learning is not simply the memorization of facts (no matter what your sixth-grade math teacher told you). Learning happens when you find a subject interesting, relevant, and meaningful. You care about it. Caring about something is not just a rational thought. Caring is an emotional behavior. I don't know about you, but the teachers I remember most are the ones who related to me, inspired me, and convinced me to care about not only the subject, but learning in general. When you care, you are driven to seek out novel experiences and information through autonomous desire. In the long run, you are driven by neither carrot nor stick but by your internal sense of meaning.

Effects of Early Experiences on Feeling States

I was raised by police officers. My mother and stepfather were police officers. Their friends were police officers. My family events, birthday parties, sports competitions, and holidays were all spent around police officers. They were my caregivers and the people who looked out for me. To this day, when I see police officers, my immediate emotional reaction is a positive one. I feel safe and pleasant. When I see an officer in uniform, I think of my mother leaving for work when I was a little boy. Logically, I understand that not all police are nice, or good, or like my parents in any way other than that they have the same job. But my bias was shaped early, so my emotional response to law enforcement is positive.

I can imagine how it might be completely different for somebody else. Like maybe their father was arrested in front of them when they were a child, and now police officers are the ones who took Dad away—the father who played with them and protected them and took care of them. Consider how that might shape a person's feeling toward law enforcement. As I write this book, I'm acutely aware of the complicated place that police officers occupy in public life today, and that's not what I'm referring to. I'm referring to the deep and lasting effect early experiences have on the algorithms that create our feeling states and how those feeling states can color our perceptions and behavior. The fact that it happens is not within our control. Everybody is subject to this biological reality. What you can do is become more aware of the feeling states that drive you in order to have a more democratic relationship with your own well-being.

Feelings Aren't Free

This brings me to an important point in this discussion about emotions: They don't exist in isolation from your physiology. Feelings aren't free. They have energetic costs in the most literal metabolic, chemical sense of the word. Surely you have had an emotionally trying day at the end of which you were exhausted. You weren't necessarily out in the forest logging trees and hauling them in on a wagon pulled by a donkey, but by God, it probably felt like it.

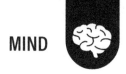

Emotional systems are directly tied into the autonomic functions discussed earlier. Experiences of joy, sadness, grief, loneliness, and anger all cost real energy. The feelings and behaviors that drive you forward place energetic demands on your physiology. That's because emotions are designed to be internal mechanisms that steer the way you engage with the world. This is powerful and necessary but can cost you big if you don't manage things well. Chronic emotional distress has known negative effects on physiology, such as elevated blood pressure and dysregulation of stress hormones like cortisol and adrenaline.

Anger, for example, is a mobilizing emotion. Feelings of anger can drive you to alter something in the environment with swift action. Anger hits the gas pedal to get you moving. That can be a powerful asset if you see something as unfair, unjust, or ethically wrong and use anger in the form of outrage to attempt to change it. It can be detrimental, however, when you smash down the physiological gas pedal because the person in front of you is driving slower than you think they should. Anger is necessary and powerful. As is compassion. As is hunger. But when misappropriated, these powerful states cost you dearly. If you can become more aware of how you relate to your internal state and have indicators for when things aren't firing in a way that serves you, you can change it.

Most of the time, this is obvious, at least when you see it in others. Things get tricky when you attempt to identify your own patterns of feeling, their origins, and the behaviors associated with them. Unfortunately, this usually doesn't occur due to a proactive approach to wellness but because the wheels start to come off the bus. Luckily (mostly), you have a beautifully evolved brain structure that helps you become aware of and modulate your baser instinctual self. When harnessed well, this part of the mind can become a wonderful asset to your well-being. When it goes astray, it can become a conspirator in narratives that cause the rationalization of bad habits and can slow your progress in the quest for performance longevity.

The Cognitive Layer

Last but not least, hitched on top of the more primal driving forces is the cognitive layer of the brain. Cognition, technically speaking, is the mental action or process of acquiring knowledge and understanding through thought, experience, and the senses. It includes functions like attention, language, learning, memory, and perception. Cognition is taking information from the rest of the physiological system and making sense of it.

Cognitive functions are executed by areas of the brain collectively referred to as the neocortex. This part of the brain conjures up images of something approximating a gray, squiggly egg. These folds allow for more surface area to develop sophisticated neural networks, creating space for the amazing cognitive functions that set humans apart from other species. While other animals express neocortical functions like speech, language, problem-solving, and social organization, they are rudimentary compared to the elaborate psychological landscape that humans experience—a double-edged sword, to say the least.

It's not within the scope of this book to dive deep into the topic of cognitive health. Experts learn more every day, and many books have been written on this important subject. We are going to fix our sights on the specific aspect that is most relevant to selecting indicators for your Performance Longevity Dashboard: executive function. Executive function is higher-order thinking characterized by decision-making, planning, abstract thought, and mental flexibility. Perhaps most importantly, it's the seat of self-control.

C-Suite Executive (The C Is for Cortex)

In recent decades, there have been rising numbers of people diagnosed with neurodegenerative disorders like Alzheimer's and dementia and attentional modulation issues like ADHD, along with increased awareness around the effects of traumatic brain injury. This, coupled with the rise of the tech entrepreneurial class and ideas like biohacking, speed-reading, and speed-learning, has created a tidal wave of interest in pumping up the octane in brain performance and, specifically, executive function.

While the expression of various executive functions often involves the cooperation of multiple areas of the brain, the frontal lobe (the area of the brain that sits behind your forehead) is thought to be the seat of these essential abilities. This collection of brain activities includes

- **Working memory:** The ability to hold on to and organize ideas that are no longer perceptually present. Think of reorganizing a to-do list or holding a thought in your head while you write something else down before you explain that thing.

- **Delayed gratification:** The ability to wait longer for the potential of a better reward versus seeking immediate gratification (getting the thing I want right now). Delayed gratification plays a major role in overcoming addiction, for example.

- **Inhibitory control:** While this does have some redundancy with delayed gratification, it refers more broadly to the ability to ignore one set of stimuli (inhibit) and drive and maintain attention where it is more relevant.

- **Creativity, cognitive flexibility, and problem solving:** While these three do have independent aspects, they have an important area of overlap: the ability to think consciously about solving novel problems. Creativity helps generate a new solution to a problem; cognitive flexibility is about seeing things from a different point of view (both literally and figuratively); and problem solving is exactly what it sounds like—the ability to seek out solutions to problems that arise in the environment, whether physical or cogitative.

- **Task switching:** This involves the ability to smoothly transition attention from one thing to another thing and use a set of skills required for one thing for another thing. Task switching, along with sustained focus and working memory, is one of the most common cognitive performance goals reported to me as a human performance practitioner.

The variety of executive functions expressed are strong predictors of life success and enjoyment. People with better executive function are less likely to commit crimes or act in unsafe ways; they are more likely to experience long-term marital harmony; and they perform predictably better at work and at school. There is way more to executive function than that, for sure. Too much to put in this book, I'll tell you that. What is most essential for our discourse is to know that there are measurable aspects to this evolutionary triumph and that these actions develop as part of both hardware and software in our brains, meaning they have a chemical, neuronal aspect to them. The chemistry of brain and body bear powerful influence over these capacities. Preventable lifestyle diseases are known contributors to cognitive decline. They are also deeply swayed by behavioral influence.

The way we use or don't use our brains can move them toward adaptive capacities that serve us well into old age or atrophy our hard-fought evolutionary benefit. Writers like Cal Newport, professor of computer science at Georgetown University and author of the book *Deep Work* (concepts from which were instrumental in the completion of this very book), have looked at the behavioral and environmental strategies we can rely on to reduce drag on our cognitive capacities to enhance cognitive performance longevity. These skills are important not just in the avoidance of disease but in an information economy increasingly dependent on thinking as a marketable skill set.

Awareness and Modulation

An interesting developmental fact is that the frontal lobe—the area of the neocortex most associated with executive function—isn't fully developed until humans reach their early twenties. This area of the brain helps you become aware of and then modulate your reactions to external stimuli. An easy example of how this plays out in everyday life is that half of the people in a work meeting probably have to pee, but nobody says a word. They just sit there, holding it. This doesn't seem amazing in a room full of adults. In fact, it's expected. But what if there was a two-year-old in that meeting? Oh boy, would everybody know that kid had to pee. Not only that, but everybody would know how they felt about having to pee, and if they had to wait too long, they might just pee their pants. That's because the part of their brain that recognizes social propriety and regulates emotion hasn't come online yet.

A two-year-old being unable to hold their pee probably isn't a novel concept, but the underlying brain physiology does have implications for the larger topics at hand. Becoming aware of what's stirring below the surface of your inner experience and then altering your behavior both in the moment and over time is a uniquely human gift often left unopened. The anterior cingulate gyrus is an especially interesting area of the brain connected to both the emotional and the cognitive areas. More and more research shows that this area is crucial in the regulation of your response to emotions. Of additional interest is that things like attention to breathing (the heart of mindfulness practices) has been shown to increase activity in this same area of the brain. More on that later.

Viktor Frankl famously said, "Between stimulus and response there is a space. In that space is our power to choose our response. In our response lies our growth and our freedom." One of the superpowers of human beings is the ability to be aware of how we are thinking, feeling, and acting and then, if we choose, to change it. My dogs go apeshit every time a package is delivered. It's all-out madness. Never in fourteen years have my dogs stopped and pondered, *Why do I feel like this? Is this a good use of my energy? How can I feel different?* This level of self-reflection is unavailable to my lovable canine companions no matter how smart I think they are. If I want them to feel and act differently toward delivery drivers, I have to be the one who alters their behavior.

Having advanced cognitive functions affords human beings lots of incredible abilities, but none is perhaps more important than to be aware of and modulate our internal state and our outward behavior. You might read that statement and think that the composure it implies means the suppression of your internal contents. As long as you act out the right steps, no harm, no foul. As discussed earlier in this chapter, unchecked internal turmoil almost always comes out in ways that are harmful, whether to yourself or to others. Even if no direct damage is done, they clutter your sensibilities and limit your ability to be flexible and adaptive in ways that ensure the expression of your best self and as a result hinder your performance longevity potential.

THE DANCE: HOW THE LAYERS OF MIND INTERACT

After discussing these basic layers of MIND and their commensurate anatomical parts in the brain, it's important to touch back on a fundamental point. That is, no one component of a system or network operates independently. There is vast interconnectivity, overlapping function, and even redundancy. The dynamic system we call the mind may not even be found in the anatomical brain alone but may be an emergent expression of the dance that is the nervous system and, if you believe in such things, the soul. Whatever your beliefs, there seems to be a uniquely human essence that emerges from the interaction of the seemingly infinite factors of our thoughts, feelings, and physiology that make us some of the most beautiful and most horrifying creatures on the planet.

The dance of the human mind can be seen in many complex behaviors that are uniquely human. For example, we are the only species that empathizes with other species. The last time I checked, no dogs were displaying handprints on their mantels in order to remember the dearly departed household human. That doesn't mean other animals don't experience loss, but they don't wrap the same level of complex behavior around it that we do. Humans are also the only animals that will fight and even die for what they believe is a righteous cause. Other animals may fight to preserve life and limb and defend territory, but they don't fight over religious beliefs or ethical differences.

Practically speaking, it is important to note that these areas of the brain are not isolated from each other because it can help us realize that homogeneous signals can indicate an array of potential issues that may need our

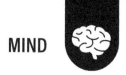

attention—the same way a check engine light on a car dashboard signals that something requires investigation. Furthermore, we can leverage that interaction to move the needle on the entire system at once. This is not only true for MIND but, as I'll cover later in the book, for the entirety of performance longevity.

The Way You Talk to Me: Cross-Communication in the Brain

The areas of the brain interweave to create the symphony that is thinking and behavior. This is true in terms of anatomical connections through synapses that cross various areas of the brain as well as functional cascades. For example, the two amygdalae have synapses that reach the hypothalamus and other structures associated with memory. This connection points to how we become conditioned to fear responses based on our experience. Conditioned fears can become more generalized over time with our wonderfully powerful imaginations weaving a web of stories that deter us from exposing ourselves to those things that make us feel afraid. Whether for legitimate protection or mere rationalization, it is clear that these structures and components of the brain do not operate in isolation. The various networks of neural circuitry coordinate to, as famed neuroscientist Andrew Huberman puts it, "play like chords on a piano." The same keys played in different combinations harmonize in unique ways that create seemingly infinite variations of sound and music.

Your emotional state can certainly affect your decision-making, problem-solving brain. The inverse is true as well. Your cognitive experience, whether it is environmental assessments or your own rumination, informs your emotional state, which can alter your physiology in real and measurable ways. This is easily provable by thinking about the possibility of erotic interaction. It's not necessary to have a partner present for the cascade of physiology to occur that prepares you for and eventually mimics the outcome of sexual intercourse. You need only imagine it. That's how powerful the connections of mind and brain are to body and experience. This doesn't happen only in the obvious example of sexual thought. Even a cursory look into the science on belief and placebo effect will astound you.

This phenomenon is not just from the top down, either. The bottom-up feedback you get from your body informs how you feel and think, too. When we describe a person who is nervous, we say that they're tense and encourage them to loosen up. We also know that posture has a powerful influence on how you feel about yourself and others, especially during social interaction. Heart rate and intensity, breathing, and muscle tension all influence your perception of your internal state and therefore the types of emotions you experience and even the types of behaviors you engage in. Ever get a "gut feeling"?

These layers of interoceptive communication that are going on every moment of every day are mind-boggling. Learning to tune in to them can be a crucial ingredient in selecting indicators for MIND. There's a vast sea of information out there on the complex topic of human neuropsychology, but one book in particular that drove it home for me was *Behave* by Robert Sapolsky, a neuroscientist and primatologist teaching at Stanford University whose work I cannot recommend highly enough. His books on human behavior are always enlightening and well written.

No topic is more evident of cross-talk or more relevant to modern life than stress. For the majority of us, life today is safer than it has ever been. We live in reliable structures, the interiors of which are kept at whatever temperature we choose. Our food is delivered to us, and we can store it in temperature-regulated cabinets for days, weeks, or even months at a time. Emergency medicine saves us from injury and infection that would have meant certain death only a century and a half ago. As true as all that is, people are stressed more than ever. This persistent stress not only places a drag on quality of life but also has a direct impact on the physiology that drives the performance of both mind and body. If left unchecked, it can also shorten your time on the road.

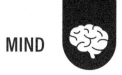

Stress: Both a Medicine and a Toxin

Stress and its negative effects have become somewhat of a boogeyman. We expend intense amounts of financial and psychological resources to avoid feeling it, be relieved from it, and manage it. In fact, this sentiment is so prevailing that the market for business stress relief was valued at somewhere between $500 million and $2.4 billion in 2022. Stress itself is not something you want to avoid, however, if such a thing were even possible. Awareness of stress, its effect on you, and ways you can modulate your reactions to it are key in learning to grow and improve from it. In so doing, you can cultivate better performance and health.

When people are asked about causes of stress, they usually report things like relationships and family, money, and work. They get piled right at the top of the list of things that can make us feel yucky. Stress is funny like that. Generally, it has a negative connotation. But stress can come from things we think of as positive, too. Graduating from college, getting married, and receiving a promotion at work are generally favorable life events, but all of them can create stress. Having a better understanding of what stress is, how it affects you, and what you can do about it is key to feeling and doing your best.

Stress in the strictest terms is any force acting on body and mind that disrupts homeostasis. When your set point for normal gets tugged on too much or pushed too far, that's stress. External factors like illness and disease as well as internal factors such as anger, loneliness, and other negative emotions can all have a direct impact on both the function of your physiology and the quality of your life.

An important and necessary part of life, short-term stress, along with the resources for rest and proper adaptation, is an ally that can actually improve your resilience. Conversely, chronic and sustained stress can overload you and lead to unwanted health outcomes as well as interfere with the expression of your potential. As biological organisms, human beings are designed to experience and respond to stress, and ideally be better prepared for it the next time. That can mean muscles getting stronger because you lift weights, or it can be better coping strategies when a family member dies.

The long-term cost of stress is referred to as "allostatic load." The accumulation of stressors in the mind and body is not simply a psychological event. Chronic stress perpetuates activation of the hormonal and autonomic stress physiology and, if not given the opportunity to reset, can result in predisposition to illness, increased mortality, and most certainly reduced performance and quality of life. These physiological states of stress can be brought about through physical action—hard sports training is an obvious example—but are also deeply intertwined with our psychological and emotional states.

At the heart of stress physiology is the body's accountant, the autonomic nervous system. The relationship between sympathetic and parasympathetic states is a constant balancing of scales. Becoming skilled at listening to and altering your autonomic state is a worthwhile effort that can yield exponential return on investment. Emotional and psychological tools are essential as well, but autonomic skills in particular are powerful and accessible levers that work with great effect and fast to help you become more adaptive. A bit later in this chapter, as well as in the workbook, we'll look at some specific examples that you can use in everyday life.

Stress can be a powerful friend and teacher. With a proper orientation, it can make you stronger and more resilient both physically and psychologically. That doesn't mean checking out or covering up its effects—just the opposite. Attuning yourself to its true consequences, both positive and negative, will help you become more skilled at being human and flowing with your changing needs as they present themselves.

SELF-REFLECTION QUESTIONS

What physical or psychological signals flash on your dashboard to let you know that you're getting too stressed?

_____

_____

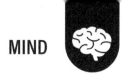

In cases where you've gotten overloaded, what indicator lights were flashing that you may have ignored?

_____

_____

Was it necessary to ignore them? Why?

_____

_____

What else could you have done to better attune yourself to that stress so you could properly adapt?

_____

_____

Of the three layers of MIND (autonomic, emotional, and cognitive), which presents the biggest challenge to you personally? What indicators might help you better tune in? What tools could you use to adjust?

_____

_____

Unsubscribe: Rocket Money for Your Brain

All of this brings me to a single relevant conclusion in regard to how the layers of MIND affect performance longevity. You have programs playing in the back of your mind without your conscious input. For the most part, being unaware of them is not only okay but actually better. Keeping things in the subconscious gives you a working map so that you can navigate life, stay safe, and meet your fundamental needs. On the other hand, you can pick up bad habits and create subtle and insidious reward systems and feedback loops that drive unwanted feelings and actions that make you less healthy physically, psychologically, and socially. This puts a drag on your energetic resources and limits your ability to be effective in the world.

It's kind of like the smartphone app Rocket Money, which links into your bank accounts and finds all of the hidden subscriptions you've had for years that are leaching money from you. The nickel-and-diming from these little subscriptions might not seem like much in a single month, but they can compound over years until one day you realize you've spent two thousand dollars on *Antique Bicycle Quarterly*. Similarly, subtle thoughts, emotions, and their related behavior loops are like little subscriptions in your subconscious. Outbursts of frustration. Dissociating during conflict. Compulsive tendencies like eating, shopping, or lying. The individual charges may not be significant, but over time they add up.

These little expenses consume energy and take money from the bank account of your health. If you have a good system for becoming more aware of these feelings and you can connect them to actions you take, then you can catch yourself in cycles of feeling, thinking, and behavior that you may not want and shift the tide. You can't unsubscribe from something you don't even know you're paying for. That's the trick when it comes to building a dashboard, isn't it? To become more aware of what it is that you are subscribing to.

Wouldn't it be nice to have a version Rocket Money, but instead of watching your bank account for insidious subscriptions, it could tell you what thoughts, feelings, and rationalizations were putting a drag on your health account? Well, there's no app for that—yet. There are, however, indicators that you can put on your Performance Longevity Dashboard to enhance your awareness of your own mind.

SELF-REFLECTION QUESTIONS

What thoughts, feelings, and actions are like running subscriptions in your mind?

_____

_____

If you decided to change them, how would you track your progress?

_____

_____

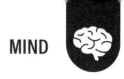

What proactive things can you do to increase the performance longevity of your mind?

_____

_____

Pick one subscription in your mind that you want to cancel.

_____

_____

Write your metric to measure your progress.

_____

_____

Pick a tool that might affect this metric. State how often you would use it and how long you would continue.

_____

_____

How will you know that you can reduce your dosage? Or do you need to do this forever?

_____

_____

WHERE IS MY MIND? INDICATORS FOR MIND

Now that you have a better understanding of some of the basic ideas of MIND, let's get practical. What I've listed in this section and the one that follows are by no means the be-all, end-all of indicators and tools that can be used to improve performance longevity in the realm of MIND. This is a subject humans have been tackling for all time. These are just examples of things that I've seen work for myself and in my career. You will experiment with some of these ideas in the workbook, too. I encourage you to give them a try now and more importantly to continue to experiment in the future. If you learn something really helpful, be sure to share it.

If you're going to take a deeper look into the layers of MIND and how they may affect your performance longevity, a good place to start is with the deepest and most far-reaching physiology we have: the autonomic nervous system. Attaching key performance indicators to this deep physiology can give you precise metrics for how well you are responding to stress. Not only that, but you can gain insight into how your behavior influences your physiology over time and take steps to improve the way you manage your life energy budget. Let's begin that journey with heart rate variability.

The Bank Statement: Heart Rate Variability

Over the last decade and a half, measuring stress resilience through the use of wearable devices has become more and more commonplace. Newly available technology allows for more direct windows into how the deepest parts of our physiology are responding to stress and how they reflect our resilience and overall well-being. The most widely used metric in this regard is heart rate variability (HRV). This metric is by no means perfect and, as I'll explain shortly, is always limited by both the hardware measuring it and the human being interpreting it. The most important thing is that learning to tune in to and alter the relationship between the gas and the brakes allows you to more actively shape your thoughts, feelings, and actions, especially in regard to how you respond to stress.

Heart rate variability is the measurement of time between heartbeats. Everybody is familiar with heart rate, which is measured in beats per minute, but many are less familiar with HRV. The time between beats of the heart is mere milliseconds, and the differences between those milliseconds are a direct reflection of whether we are pressing more on the gas pedal or more on the brakes. More sympathetic activity (gas) is marked by not just a predictable increase in heart rate but also a reduction in variability. When your body senses stress, whether it's from acute exercise or an emotionally challenging conversation, your heart rate increases and becomes more regular. Parasympathetic activity (brakes) is marked by a decrease in heart rate and an increase in HRV. Measuring heart rate variability on an ongoing basis can give you insight into how well you are responding to stress by showing you when and what pushes the gas pedal and, perhaps more important, how capable you are at pumping the brakes so that you can reset, heal, and adapt to those stressors (allostasis).

Remember, stress in and of itself is not bad. Exercise is stress. Getting married is stress. Traveling for a work opportunity is stress. A better and more sophisticated way to think of it might be: How much does this cost? Using metrics like HRV is like reviewing a bank statement. You don't want to fixate on a few dollars' difference from day to day (unless you've only got a few dollars in there to begin with!). What's more pertinent is understanding your "stress budget." If you know your budget, then you can make good decisions about when to spend and when to save.

That brings to me to an important point that speaks directly to some of the concepts discussed in Chapter 2. When you begin to track data points for health, it's easy to get hyper-focused on absolute values represented by "high" and "low" HRV scores—measures of performance. Don't. Instead, understand what it is you are really trying to change: measures of effectiveness. Do you care that the number on the app is higher, or do you care that the number on the app gives you insight into how you're feeling and operating in life? Pay attention to how your numbers trend over time and which behaviors cause changes for the better and which ones make things worse.

Using this metric is something we'll explore in some of the Personal Health Experiments in the workbook. That said, heart rate variability is by no means the only indicator of autonomic activity or your reaction to stress, so don't worry if you don't have access to a wearable device that measures HRV. There are other ways access this information that, while not quite as direct, are good enough to learn from and make decisions that encourage performance longevity.

Know Thyself: Emotional Scales and Personality Tests

Your emotional state can be much harder to pin down into numeric values than your autonomic physiology. Even though it can be trickier to measure, there are a variety of emotional scales that use questionnaires to develop statistically reliable measures of emotional experience and intelligence. These tools are most often used in research and therapeutic environments but can be helpful for developing clarity about your own emotional tendencies.

Personality tests can be another helpful resource to inform your dashboard. While some can seem like hokey party tricks, others have been developed through rigorous scientific research. The most widely used is probably the Big Five Personality Inventory. As I mentioned in the introduction to this book, the Big Five defines five personality traits: Openness, Conscientiousness, Extraversion, Agreeableness, and Neuroticism (collected under the acronym OCEAN). Each of these traits is further subdivided into two components in which you are assigned percentile scores.

While "tests" like these can help you develop insight into your personal tendencies, do not be tempted to use this type of resource to rationalize behavior that hurts yourself or others. With that said, I've found it very helpful for both myself and the clients I work with to bolster emotional strengths and reveal weaknesses. In order to accomplish this, you must first "know thyself," as Plato so aptly put it in the fourth century BC.

Pad and Pen: Journaling

Another helpful strategy for gaining insight into your emotional layer is writing. I don't mean writing a to-do list. I'm talking about stream-of-consciousness, free-flowing writing. This can be done in a diary or journal of some sort and does not necessarily need to be structured, although it seems like there are roughly two billion self-help journals on the market these days. I've used a few, and they can be insightful. Which one works for you will probably be driven primarily by aesthetics, so try some out and see what you like. What matters is that the journal you choose encourages you to truly self-reflect.

One writing exercise that I have found quite helpful is Morning Pages from Julia Cameron's book *The Artist's Way.* Every morning, you open up a notebook and write three pages about whatever you want. Multiple people I trust recommended this practice to me before I finally went for it. For some—and I was certainly in this camp—journaling and most other writing tools seem like a silly form of catharsis reserved for preteen girls. But I was once again proven wrong. Writing has been shown to improve mental health, especially when you are trying to reconcile emotionally impactful experiences.

The writing you do does not have to be specifically focused on a cathartic outcome, but the act of writing seems to clear the cobwebs from thinking and forces you to articulate your feelings. When you do so, it's an opportunity to take a beat and ask yourself, *Is that how I really feel? Why? Do I want to feel like this? How do I change it?*

Friends and Family Plan: Relationships

It's easy to get fooled by your own internal perception of how you're doing. Relying on your personal opinion as the sole source of your status is not only a way to write your own ticket to delusion, but also a massive lost opportunity to rely on communal wisdom and perspective. There is some truth to the old gentlemen's joke, "How do you know if you're in a bad mood? Your wife tells you." You can get so entrenched in feedback loops of feeling, mood, and habit that you often don't realize how you are expressing your feelings until somebody tells you directly or through their behavioral response to you.

Neither the indications nor the consequences of your emotional state exist in a vacuum. For this set of emotional indicators for your dashboard, you're going to steer away from things you do alone and consider relationship indicators. Your emotions and their behavioral outcomes have direct impacts not only on your internal state but also on how you relate to others. Your ability to form lasting and meaningful social connections is a direct consequence of emotional context, and as such, relationships can serve as a flare gun that lets you know where you truly stand.

The easiest access point for many is family. Parents, siblings, and spouses spend the most time with you and thus have the most potential to offer you feedback about how your emotional state is affecting your behavior. Whether it's through direct communication or through the emotional patterns that only family can evoke, you can get insight into what drives your deepest feeling states and think about whether those states are the ones you want to choose for yourself moving forward.

Therapeutic relationships like those with a mentor, therapist, counselor, or religious leader can also be resources for perspective, although these people may not have as much access to you as a spouse, partner, or dear friend would. The caveat of course is that you must be forthcoming about your authentic emotional state—which can be difficult to articulate and downright scary to share. It's important to surround yourself with a circle of loved ones, friends, and advisors who listen and will give you helpful and honest feedback while acting in good faith.

People who are close to you and care for you can help bring patterns that don't serve you to your awareness so you can improve. Just as important, they can encourage and support you when you are offering your best. How much stock gets put into the words and feelings of others certainly differs from one individual to another. Not everybody has your best interest in mind, so fixating on the opinions of others can become its own issue. One thing remains clear, though: No person is an island. If you are totally disconnected from social feedback, your thoughts, feelings, and behaviors will almost assuredly go astray. Just be sure to choose your company wisely.

While certainly imperfect, attending to cues from those close to you and the way you act out your internal states in the world are essential indicators to include as you build the MIND portion of your dashboard. To that end, there are questions you can ask yourself that will point you in the right direction. I go into more detail in the workbook, but here's a good question to start with:

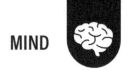

Do I have obvious and easily identifiable relationships with people around me who I feel care about me and are willing to communicate with me honestly and in good faith?

I truly hope you do. Those people, while also certainly struggling with the smudges on their own lenses, can be an integral part of identifying behaviors that are unproductive and potentially detrimental to your health and performance. One of the benefits of long-standing friendships and even monogamous partners is that those people see your trends for better or worse, and if you are mutually committed to each other's development, they may express to you hindrances that you might otherwise be unaware of or afraid to face.

SELF-REFLECTION QUESTIONS

Can you think of a situation where you ignored indicators related to MIND?

_____

_____

Were you unaware of the indicator, did you interpret it incorrectly, or did you just ignore it?

_____

_____

What happened as a result?

_____

_____

DEVELOPING IN-SIGHT: TOOLS FOR MIND

Tuning in to your internal states of MIND can be difficult. Noise from the external world tends to blend together with your internal perceptions, habits, and emotional reactions to disrupt the clarity of the signals you receive. While people like to think that the noise of the human mind is particular to their time and generation, it is not. That's why human beings have been developing cultural performance technologies and their associated mindsets for these issues for millennia. Think tai chi from China or yoga from India. Modern science can help us better explain and more precisely calibrate these technologies, but I assure you, humans have been humaning for as long as humans have existed. That's good news because it means there are proven and, to my delight, proximal strategies for learning to tune brain and mind to receive better internal information. Let's explore a few that can be useful additions to your Performance Longevity Toolkit. You'll have opportunities to try some of these tools using the Personal Health Experiments in the workbook as well.

Mindfulness 2.0

In Western culture, mindfulness and its associated forms of meditation and therapy have only been a part of common parlance since the mid-twentieth century, when the hippie revolution brought Eastern traditions to the forefront. These strategies for self-reflection hearken back far further to meditation traditions rooted in Hinduism and Buddhism. While yoga has been co-opted by sticky mats and stretch pants in North America, its true purpose is to identify blocks to a clear mind and eliminate them through the practice of various forms of exercise and meditation.

Mindfulness meditations and therapies involve turning attention inward to foster awareness of the thoughts, feelings, and behaviors that you maintain and how they may be affecting feeling states of your body. They can also include biofeedback, where technological devices like heart rate monitors or even an EEG (electroencephalogram) measuring brainwaves can give you real-time feedback as you take an internal inventory and apply

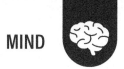

tools and interventions to alter how you think and feel. This is connecting your executive functions to your emotional systems with focused attention. (Remember that anterior cingulate thingy?) Mindfulness teachers who hail from Buddhist traditions, such as Jon Kabat Zinn and Thich Nhat Hanh, teach that mindfulness can be explored through partitioned daily practices where you sit quietly and execute specific exercises like breathing protocols or integrated into everyday behaviors like washing dishes. In either case, they can help you become a more skilled arbiter of your internal life.

"Rest Is Not Idleness"

Purposeful awareness practices have long been part of humankind, but untethered daydreaming is perhaps even older. It turns out that setting aside time to allow your mind to wander can help you reconcile experiences and emotions to make better sense of what the heck is going on in this existential mess called living and breathing. The beautifully written paper "Rest Is Not Idleness," by Mary Helen Immordino-Yang, et al., describes how downtime that allows the mind to wander is essential for health and learning.

Much of mental performance and health is focused on initiatives related to increasing attention and task orientation—things that point your mind outward into the world. But it turns out that the activities of brain and mind during awake but diffuse attention are essential for psychological and emotional performance longevity as well. During mentally unstructured activities like daydreaming, areas of the brain associated with the default mode network are activated. This network improves and maintains abilities such as abstract thought that, rather than introducing new knowledge, help connect and contextualize old memories and new information into understanding, improve social emotions like empathy and admiration, and even have implications for the development of morality.

The development of laserlike focus is not mutually exclusive from resting states of the brain. The current model represents the skill of purposefully transitioning between states of outward and internal focus. Focused attention followed by purposeful relaxation is a clear pathway to maintaining neuroplasticity (the brain's ability to change) and learning over the long haul. This is an important place to take note of how much modern technology is fighting to keep us externally focused. I'm not in the "technology is bad" camp; it's helpful, and I use it. If it weren't for social media, my career would not have developed in the way that it did. However, it is necessary to recognize what a stranglehold these tools can have on your attention even when you are not directly interacting with them. To that end, it can be important to build in time for mental rest and reflection. There will be opportunities to explore this idea through personal experimentation in the workbook.

Shoshin: Beginner's Mind

As cliché as it may seem, old dogs learning new tricks keeps those dogs young in mind. A commitment to learning new things has measurable positive effects on the mind, brain, and body as well as offers opportunities to develop emotional resilience. Shoshin, a Japanese Zen concept, means "beginner's mind." This mindset is grounded in humility and a willingness to learn, but in my experience, it has broader implications for the performance longevity of our minds.

Exposing yourself to novel situations, especially in environments in which you are unsure of the outcome, forces you to stretch your knowledge, your emotions, and, as it turns out, the physical structure and chemistry of your brain, too. When you willfully expose yourself to a new learning situation, you have the opportunity be vulnerable—to admit that you don't know what to do. One place I've seen this play out a hundred times is on the jiu-jitsu mat. The skill gap between even a moderately seasoned practitioner of grappling and a person new to the art is difficult to explain to those who have not experienced it. There is no dose of humility quite like being held down against your will by another adult. Whether it comes in the form of signing up for jiu-jitsu lessons, taking up pickleball, or enrolling in a pottery class, putting yourself into a new environment for the purpose of keeping up the ability to learn is a good thing.

My friend Zee Durham, a former Green Beret and a black belt in jiu-jitsu, likes to say, "Exposure equals composure." That's not just an awesome catchphrase; it's the truth. Composure is not the denial of emotional reality. Suppression usually results in a loss of composure in the least opportune moments. Instead, real composure is about being attuned to the psychological and emotional reality underneath the surface and having the skills of self-possession to remain calm in spite of them. It's one of the important differences between humans and our beastly cousins. It's the most important distinction between maturity and callowness. Trying new things gives us a practical road to the maintenance of our composure muscles.

You may be wondering, *What exactly does shoshin have to do with performance longevity of the mind?* Lots. As you age, and more precisely, as you become competent at navigating your own little world, your mind can become stale. You bump into fewer challenges that push your brain into growth. I mean this in the most literal sense. Effortful learning of new things as an adult has been shown to increase neurogenesis (the growth of new neural connections) in areas of the brain associated with memory and even the ways in which we pursue and perceive rewards. An absence of effortful learning and emotional challenge causes the brain and mind to atrophy.

The concept of shoshin doesn't necessarily provide information about how to expand your cognitive and emotional abilities in a literal sense. What it does is open room to purposefully engage in a continual process of learning. By adopting the mindset of a humble beginner, you can improve your access to performance longevity in profound ways. During the challenges of learning, take note of the mental and emotional struggles that arise and ask yourself questions such as these:

- What strategies do I have to deal with negative emotions if they come up?
- How well can I retain and apply information? Do I have a strategy for doing so?
- How do I interact with my peers in the learning environment?
- Am I willing to ask for help?

- How do I deal with struggle?

These are all valid and helpful questions that not only help you learn the material you may be studying but in effect perpetuate your ability to learn altogether.

I Don't Need Sunny Skies: Outdoor Activity

Actually, you do need sunny skies.

All of the biohacks, nootropics, and brain games in the world are not as reliable for improving cognitive and emotional performance and longevity as simply going outside. Time in nature has been shown to improve working memory and sustained attention as well as reduce emotional stress, anxiety, and depression. The great outdoors provides opportunity to move the body and use the mind in the way nature intended: to navigate challenges in the natural world. As it turns out, returning to that from which we came, albeit in more controlled conditions, massively benefits our mental and emotional well-being.

Some studies show as little as fifty minutes of outdoor time per day can improve cognitive function, especially for those who are already vulnerable. In one interesting study using EEG, both sitting and walking outdoors were shown to improve attention restoration and reduce rumination (repetitive negative thoughts). There is strong evidence that programs revolving around outdoor activities such as fishing, hunting, and surfing dramatically improve post-traumatic stress symptoms in veteran populations.

There are certainly confounding variables when it comes to the exact mechanisms of improvement derived from time spent outside. Is it that you have time away from the devices that zap you of your vital cognitive resources? Or is it that the outdoors inspires natural forms of exercise, like walking, hiking, and climbing? Is the power of the sun raising your vitamin D levels and signaling your brain for more complete rest? It's probably all of them to some degree. If you're in a lab writing a research paper, mechanisms matter. If your goal is a net positive in the pursuit of performance longevity,

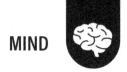

then these overlapping components are something to be exploited. Now go outside and play with your friends.

IF YOU DON'T MIND, IT DOES MATTER

The performance longevity of our minds and brains is a topic of constant conversation in all things health and fitness. As it should be. Just like the more concrete parts of your being that are the subjects of the next two chapters, you need indicators of performance for what's going on in your mind as well as some warning lights to let you know when things start to slide a bit too far. As you continue, I want to highlight that MIND is woven together with the other categories in the M3 Model.

Later, when we begin to explore the practical application of your dashboard and toolkit through the experimental mindset, we'll take a look at how the components of the M3 Model are tied together. Loss of mobility and chronic pain have a major influence on mood and quality of life, for example. Sleep loss (in terms of both quality and quantity) can have a dramatic effect on your mental and emotional well-being, too. Just ask any overtired three-year-old at bedtime on Christmas day. (Adults aren't much better, by the way; we're just more adept at rationalizing and compensating for it.)

Indicators from one category can and often do influence things in another. After all, we are but one unified system. By building a dashboard and continuously testing your indicators and tools, you can become more aware of what's going on internally so you can change the oil before the engine seizes.

What I've just presented is a cursory explanation of three metaphorical layers of MIND. Human neuropsychology is incredibly complex and gives rise to a vast amount of behavior and probably incalculable variations in internal life. It's one of the things that make people interesting. The point isn't to provide you with a literal representation of the anatomy and physiology of your neural network or a map of your psychological landscape.

Instead, the goal is to realize that it's essential to bring a higher degree of awareness to how your internal life and outward behavior affect each other in subtle and important ways. Furthermore, if you can develop clear indicators for your mind, then you can stay ahead of issues that can cause big trouble. This is true whether you're trying to maintain memory as you age, deal with stress more constructively, or develop a deeper connection in a relationship.

It's easy for things that seem small and innocuous to slip from your consciousness and become insidious little seeds that grow into devilish trees. This brings us right back to where we started: the check engine light on that dashboard. What indicator lights could help you maintain a better sense of what's going on under the hood? What tools reliably move the needle to steer you back toward a balanced state? I've shared some examples that have stood the test of time and are backed by research. It's imperative that you try things out for yourself to find what works best for you. Be sure to check out the Personal Health Experiments for MIND located in the workbook.

"Someone who is searching feels or sees things long before other people do. He or she develops a special insight, a particular kind of sensitivity. We should see this positively—this insight or sensitivity can be as useful as a warning light in a car. It tells us that there is something wrong and we would be wise to find out what it is."

—T. K. V. Desikachar, *The Heart of Yoga*

STRESS MARKERS

I met Client H when he was in high school. His parents brought him into my massage therapy clinic to help him recover from chronic shin splints that were going to take him out of his senior year of football. With some manual therapy and some simple stretches, he was back in action in short order. That's not what this particular story is about, though. H and I stayed in touch over the course of the next fifteen years and worked together on all sorts of health- and performance-related projects, from preparing for Golden Gloves boxing (which he won) all the way to getting healthy for television and film roles.

H is by far one of the most tenacious, driven, and hardworking human beings I have ever met. If Type A personality had a poster child, H would be the toothy thumbs-up guy on that poster. For the most part, it has served him well. Against all odds, H has built a robust career in the entertainment industry, an industry in which the chance of success is as statistically close to zero as one can possibly get. As with many Type A people, along with the robust determination comes a lack of ability to relax.

For H, this can express itself as anxiety, restlessness, and serious sleep disruption—all things that he, at least at first, accepted as part and parcel of working incredibly hard. To be honest, sometimes they are. At least in small doses. However, when it becomes part of a larger dishevelment, like it did for Client H, it becomes a problem. H started experiencing mood disruptions, malaise, demotivation, fatigue, chronic nagging injuries, and even an increase in nervous tics. All this in an otherwise healthy, fit young man.

When H and I talked about it, at first he wasn't aware of where these things were coming from. To him, they sort of showed up out of the blue. But by this point in the book, you know better, don't you? As H and I pulled on the thread, he realized that there had been little signs that he hadn't connected to his current state. To him, the pain, fatigue, and emotional disruption were, quite honestly, obstacles to be hurdled in pursuit of his professional goals. With practice and maturity, H has gotten better at identifying signals earlier and using tools to course-correct when he needs to.

Being tough as hell only gets you so far, and it does not have to be mutually exclusive with self-care. Would anybody argue that buying a really well-built car is a reason not to perform regular maintenance on it? Well-built just means that it will tolerate more of your crap before it shuts down, not that abusing it will make it run better. The same goes for humans. Even the toughest among us have fundamental operating needs that, when met, allow for sustained performance over the long haul.

> **"** *Most of what goes on within us remains dulled and hidden from us until it reaches the muscles."*
>
> —**Moshe Feldenkrais,** *Awareness Through Movement*

CHAPTER 5: | MVMT

My family hails from Buffalo, New York, where the yearly average snowfall is just shy of 70 inches. Nestled around Lake Erie, Buffalo is known for harsh winters and rapid weather changes. For example, a couple years ago around Thanksgiving, my grandmother went to sleep with the ability to see her grass and woke up in the morning unable to open the doors to her house.

Due to this abundant snowfall and the erratic nature of the winter climate in general, everybody in Buffalo knows you have to wash your car on a regular basis in wintertime. Local municipalities salt the roads constantly to melt ice, and the slush splashes up onto your vehicle as you travel those roads. Over time, the salt can cause massive amounts of rust and destroy your car.

Can you drive your car without washing it? Sure. But eventually the oxidation will eat holes in the trunk, muffler, doors, and floorboards. Factually speaking, your car *can* work without those parts, but eventually the decay will get into something that really matters. If you want your vehicle to run as well as it can, you've got to keep it clean. The same goes for your joints, muscles, and tissues. The abuse of life, injury, and misuse accumulates. If you don't have good systems of care for your body, it may not fall to pieces in a single moment of failure, but one thing is for sure: You won't get everything out of that marvel of biology that you otherwise could.

WAITING GAME

"I used to be able to" is the battle cry of a lagging indicator gone awry. When you don't regularly and purposefully test the borders of your physicality, you are putting blinders on in regard to your ability to move through the world.

Much of the time, we don't know that something is going wrong until we have lost functionality or pain starts to detract from our quality of life. And pain is a big problem. Back pain is the number one reason people visit their primary care physician, and chronic pain accounts for $635 billion in annual healthcare costs in the U.S. Not to mention the connection between these figures and the epidemic of addiction occurring with pain relief medications.

Our success in generating convenience via technological advancement is creating a movement-impoverished culture in which the general public is less and less physically capable and more and more fragile and pain-ridden. An ever-decreasing connection to our physical environment begins a loop of frailty and avoidance that limits exploration of and engagement with our surroundings as well as reduces our ability to participate in important social conventions. Even the slightest increase in awareness has the potential to open the door to better living and performance.

Relying solely on lagging indicators to guide your behaviors regarding the maintenance and course-correction of the body progressively narrows the options you have to navigate your environment. Waiting around for pain and/or loss of function is like waiting for your car's engine to catch fire before you add coolant. Markers like grip strength, foot speed, and the ability to get up and down off the ground without using your hands (all leading indicators of fall risk) are well-known links to all-cause mortality and can be helpful indicators on your MVMT dashboard. I am aware of the fundamental truth that, yes, things fall apart. The human body doesn't last forever any more than an automobile does. However, the certainty of finality does not have to include the certainty of decrepitude. What's more, preventing the latter does not need to be complicated. Applying simple, reliable systems for movement will provide information about functionality, let you know when

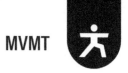

it's time to perform maintenance and basic repairs, and point you toward more effective tools to achieve those ends.

As I've discussed throughout this book, just as you should install smoke detectors before the house catches fire, you should have valid, reliable, accessible indicators for when trouble is brewing in your muscles and joints. Smoke detectors for movement, if you will. In this chapter, we're going to look at some of these smoke detectors for human movement. We'll consider some basic ideas about how movement is organized as well as ways you can maintain your grip on your movement capacity over time (pun intended). We'll take lessons from some of my colleagues at the tip of the spear in sports performance and examine how those same concepts can help anybody who wants to move and feel better. Additionally, we'll explore how you can apply those ideas to your Performance Longevity Dashboard as well as some tools you can experiment with that I've found effective as both a coach and a person trying to stay strong and mobile so I can perform at my best.

WHY DO WE MOVE?

"Why do we move?" is kind of a funny question to ask because the answer seems so obvious. We move to get around the world and stuff, right? To get things we need and do things we want to do. Sure, on some level that's true. But let's be more specific. Why does any organism move? Biologically, there are two reasons: to move away from threats (things that are potentially harmful and may limit its chances to produce offspring) and to pursue opportunities (things that keep it alive and improve its chances to produce offspring). As animals explore their habitats, environmental obstacles present themselves that challenge their ability to do these very things. Any organism's ability to adapt movement solutions to a broad range of problems in their environment is a direct indication of their health. This is true whether the problem is a busted dorsal fin or it's that you can't carry your groceries up the stairs without sweating buckets or busting a knee.

The ability to avoid threats and pursue opportunities isn't just an abstract piece of movement biology, either. Threats can mean the obvious evolutionary examples of avoiding predators and environmental catastrophes (think fleeing a pack of hungry wolves or getting out of dodge when a tornado comes). Less obvious threats are the pain, dysfunction, and disease that can come from being movement malnourished. The same goes for the opportunity side of the house. Yes, seeking and competing for mates, shelter, and food resources are a part of the evolutionary function of movement. But more human than that, the ability to move well affords us opportunities to more thoroughly engage with life. We are freer to express ourselves, whether it happens to be in the performance of a sport, dancing at family celebrations, or maintaining independence and functionality as we age.

MOVEMENT INTELLIGENCE

Movement intelligence is the ability to coordinate your body and manipulate objects in space and time. This *kinesthesia* is made up of the trifecta of proprioceptive, vestibular, and visual sensory systems, each with its own special contributions to our larger movement capacity.

- The proprioceptive sense comes from nerves embedded in joints and soft tissues. These proprioceptors provide feedback that help you determine how much motion you can express at these segments and at which speeds and directions.

- The vestibular system is in the inner ear and is responsible for spatial orientation and balance. The canals of the inner ear sense the position of your head in space and work with the other components as a sort of gyroscope to orient your feeling of which way is up.

- The visual system is the orientation of your eyes to determine your place and the place of objects in space and time. Your eyes play an essential role in spatial orientation as well as the calculation of movement of the body and your response to objects in the environment.

These three aspects syngerize to form kinesthesia. As is often the case with biology, these three components offer redundancies in forming your movement map so that if one goes down, the other two can and will pick up the slack. (For example, if you get some sawdust in your eyes while you're sanding your hardwood floors, you don't just fall over. Your other senses help pick up the burden, albeit with some hindrance.)

The development of kinesthesia is a normal part of biological development. We move through whatever habitat we might find ourselves in as we mature from newborns and infants to toddlers, children, adolescents, and adults. We progress from simple oral and tactile experience to visual and auditory/vestibular experience. Then later we crawl, walk, run, climb, and jump. During this process, we develop many of our default habits for moving, and so the broader our movement exposure during these highly impressionable periods of development is, the more robust our movement capacity tends to be.

I was fortunate to have been exposed to a wide variety of movement education as a kid. I took swim lessons and went to surf camp, practiced martial arts starting at around age six, played baseball, and even got exposed to resistance training as early as age eleven or twelve. Our garage never had cars in it. We had heavy bags, skateboards, roller skates, surfboards and body boards, nets for soccer and hockey, various exercise gadgets, and much more. I believe this variety of exposure and opportunity for movement played a large role in my continued health to this day.

The caveat to all of that is no matter how vast your movement experience is early in life, it can go away. Easily. Not only that, but sometimes when you get it early and don't maintain it, you can fall into a trap of delusion about your current capacity. This is where the "hold my beer" challenge moments go wrong, and Dad tears his groin at the family barbecue because he thinks he can still do the splits after all these years.

These highly adaptable sensorimotor capacities in humans have evolved over millions of years to help us better solve problems that present themselves in whatever environments we might find ourselves in. The appreciation for the capacity to solve problems creatively is on display in the way we celebrate sports and idolize athletes. The oohs, aahs, and never-ending sports highlight reels show our intrinsic appreciation for the ability to move well and solve environmental problems. Especially when those things are done under challenging conditions. Your capacity for motion is not just for the sake of sports performance, though. The ability to navigate problems in your environment is a sliding scale. Most of us will never dunk a basketball, sprint across the finish line at the Olympics, or throw a baseball at ninety miles per hour. Being a capable human being who can express basic movement patterns with vigor and efficiency has proven over and over again not only to predict longevity at the highest levels of performance but also to predict levels of basic life performance in general.

When it comes to the preservation of movement, many people aim to simply continue to perform to the narrow task demands of the life they are accustomed to. But it's not the expected and the well practiced that gets us. It's the slow degradation of capacity that makes us vulnerable to challenges we did not anticipate. If you have exactly enough money coming in to pay your bills every month with nothing left over and no savings, is that financial robustness? Of course not. If your car suddenly needs repairs or you need a new washing machine, you will be broke. It works the same way when it comes to managing the movement capacity of your body. Moreover, most people don't even have a real sense of how much is in the account until there's no more money. Better to build a reserve of capacity—a savings account—so that if you are called upon for more, whether for emergency or enjoyment, you can meet those demands with vigor.

This chapter and the corresponding personal health experiments are all about tuning in to the current condition of your movement intelligence, assigning valid, reliable, accessible indicators to help keep track of your movement, and using appropriate tools to keep things in working order.

RANGE OF MOVEMENT

It is a readily accepted fact that we have vital signs for health that should be within certain ranges. If you go to your doctor for a checkup, getting your blood pressure taken is a normal part of the process. When you do, they compare you to other people of the same age, gender, and ethnicity. These normative values (the range of what's expected in a population) let them know if your blood pressure is too low, too high, or just right. Imagine if you were way out of the normative range, teetering on hypertension and cardiovascular disease. What would happen? Recommended changes in lifestyle and maybe even a prescription for medication. Action would be taken to restore you to normal range. Rightfully so.

Well, your chemistry is not the only thing that has acceptable ranges. Your movement has acceptable ranges, too. People say things like, "My range of motion in my hips isn't so good. I can't really bend over anymore," with a tone of blanket acceptance. Can you imagine leaving your blood pressure unchecked? There'd be serious consequences. The same is true for your ability to move your body well. It's important to have vital signs for movement that speak to how well you can navigate the demands of life. Do you need the abilities of a Cirque du Soleil contortionist or an Olympic wrestler to achieve performance longevity? Not at all. The noble pursuit of better movement, however, will improve your ability not just to exist longer but to live and perform better.

When we look at indicators for the movement of the human body, range of motion usually refers to the amount of movement that is available at a given joint or in a larger movement, like a squat. It is usually measured in numerical degrees of freedom by a tool like a goniometer. While this chapter focuses on range of motion, it is by no means the only essential attribute in determining movement quality. Attributes like coordination (the ability of various muscles to work together to produce a desired movement), agility (the ability to slow down, speed up, or change direction), and balance (the ability to maintain or return your center of mass over your base of support) all play similarly important roles in how well you move. Think of these attributes as bands on a stereo equalizer. Based on your genetics and your collection of life experiences, these bands will be at different levels.

In my experience, range of motion has the greatest ability to limit the other attributes and reduce the freedom needed to support performance in work, sport, and life.

ORGANIZING MOTION

The human physical structure is remarkably adaptable. It only takes a quick trip to a public park or shopping mall to see the incredible variety of problem-solving that occurs in order to continue ambulation in spite of severe obesity, injury, postural distortion, or congenital anomaly.

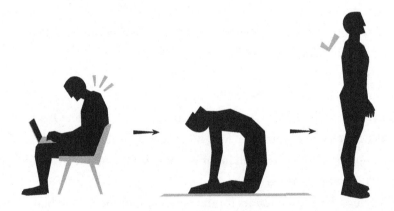

The tolerance for potential malfunctions, whether they originate from the inside out or vice versa, is deep, wide, and impressive. We are made to keep on keeping on. *The human body is an incredible machine capable of continued adaptation, for better or for worse.* Adaptive mechanisms can take place that are not for ensuring performance longevity but instead are unconscious responses to demands placed on your structure. For there to be a predictably positive outcome that contributes to performance longevity, you have to more fully participate in the direction of your own adaptive processes. Ultimately, the accumulation of unchecked insults over time will reduce your bandwidth of available movement solutions and blunt your ability to adapt in the future.

If the goal is to organize a dashboard that gives you reliable information about how much and how well you can move at any given time, then it's helpful to understand two categorical differences in how we think about movement in general: task completion strategies and formal movement strategies. While these two strategies don't by any means fully cover the vast complexity that organizes human motion, they do provide a useful way to think about how you move so that you can pay closer attention to what the heck you are doing and develop better ways to stay ahead of the curve.

Everybody Hurts

Along with exploring formal indicators for movement and tools to improve it, it's important to discuss one of the biggest limiters in our capacity to move well: pain.

Pain is a strange bird. It is not so much a thing as it is an experience. Pain can be caused by physical mechanisms like neurological damage, tissue inflammation, organ distress, and chronic disease states. It can also be influenced by less tangible but equally powerful mental and emotional states. Stress, anxiety and depression, trauma, and beliefs about pain (including both personal experience and culture) all influence your relationship with pain. In the absence of obvious catastrophic injury or insult, the onset of pain is multifactorial in nature and so often includes multiple contributing factors. All of this to say that our basic biology is made to drive our attention to alleviating pain for lots of reasons. While the alleviation of pain is an important part in maintaining your ability to move well, it is not necessarily a valid indicator of your potential for movement.

Because pain is a subjective experience, the best we can do to measure it, unfortunately, is to ask a person about their experience. Not a lot to go on. When I was working in the realm of return to play and therapeutics, improvements in felt experience were certainly important, but indicators such as the tendency to withdraw from stimulation and avoid movement were often more reliable signs of improvement.

Think of limping after you sprain your ankle or wincing when you grab the jug of milk out of the fridge with the arm that has tendonitis. While these things should not be ignored entirely, they are often a small part of a much bigger picture. The causes of pain and discomfort are many, and the alleviation of pain is usually but a first step in the longer process of moving toward a more robust capacity to move. Focusing on pain relief alone is like putting tape over your dashboard so that you can't see the flashing check engine light anymore.

Subjective experience is important, but not without being calibrated against more objective key performance indicators (KPIs) that can further validate or challenge your internal sense of things. Next, we'll take a look at a simple way to organize the movement of your body so you can become a more aware and educated participant in the direction of your movement evolution.

PAIN IS LOW RESOLUTION

Client S might be one of my most interesting clients ever. Their care required lots of flexibility and creativity and forced me to think outside the box of how I might normally render service to a pain relief client. S came to my clinic with a primary complaint of trauma-induced neuropathic shoulder pain. The trauma was a kick from a horse that for all intents and purposes exploded S's shoulder joint. And that's not all. S also had a history of multiple head traumas as well as botched medical care that resulted in a distrust of providers. Not a great starting line. In spite of all that, one thing was clear: S was motivated to improve the experience of their body in both feel and function.

Due to S's suspicious bent and intolerance for movement variability, it took some time to explore the options for rebuilding capacity. A minor insult to the system could create debilitating pain that lasted for days. This repetitive experience of crushing and demotivating pain caused S to close the window of available movement strategies and over time essentially blunt bodily communication to the binary toggle of pain/no pain. On one hand, avoiding pain-inducing movement makes total sense. Avoid new insults to the system so things don't get worse. However, closing the aperture on movement solutions often begets a myth of frailty that undermines the remarkable potential for improved robustness given the proper conditions.

After some experimentation, we found some basic exercises that S could handle, but regardless of any temporary success that any exercise yielded, one important limitation remained: S's primary marker of movement was still based in whether or not they were experiencing pain. Pain, while an essential biological indicator, is a vague one. The lens of pain for human movement is like looking through smudged glasses. You get some sense of what's happening, but the details are fuzzy.

In addition to being locked into pain as a primary indicator, S displayed some psychological hang-ups when performing what they viewed as physical therapy–type exercises since they'd failed to yield results and even worsened symptoms in the past. The hang-ups weren't so much about the efficacy of the exercises themselves but rather that they wouldn't lead to anywhere productive and would only serve as a reminder of things S could no longer do. So I was confronted with a problem as a practitioner: What could I offer S that would help them attune to their body in a meaningful way, inspired actionable self-care, and didn't invoke familiarity with a failed plan?

Somehow I landed on Filipino stick fighting. I'm not kidding. I grew up doing various martial arts, one of which was Kali, a Filipino stick and knife fighting discipline. While I abandoned the practice of Kali in my late teens, I maintained some of the basic movements as part of my exercise repertoire. They challenge the shoulder, elbow, and wrist in fun and interesting ways that just aren't possible with free weights. I introduced these basic motions to S on a hunch, and wouldn't you know it, they became obsessed with it, engaging in at-home practice, watching tutorial videos in their free time, and traveling to seminars. Kali became a central part of S's life.

What does all this have to do with movement indicators and the development of a toolkit for improving the experience of bodily motion? Well, rather than having a limited language of pain-or-no-pain, S could get higher-resolution feedback including which angles, speeds, weights, and contexts improved or degraded their ability to perform the motions of this martial art. Is Kali representative of normative value in human motion in the strictest sense of the term? No. Did it provide S with a truer representation of their potential movement capacity? Absolutely.

Along with that, it has motivated S to pursue new health behaviors that support their ability to continue to participate in this hobby. "I exercise because I want to be able to _____ " can be a helpful anchor to have in place to keep the boat from floating too far away. You don't listen to the engine and check the oil in your car simply for the sake of doing it. You do it so you know if that vehicle will perform for you in the ways that are meaningful to you.

Task Completion

Task completion is exactly what it sounds like—completing a task or set of tasks. Over the years, I've asked lots of my students and clients what they think of when I ask them about moving the body with a task completion strategy. "Get 'er done," "Just do it," and "Do the damn thing" are common answers. To prod them further, I ask what situations might fit into this category. Military and other tactical professionals offer answers like boot camp and (special forces) selection, fighting, mission completion, medical emergencies, arresting a suspect, and fighting a fire. Correctamundo. I also get simpler answers like walking to your car, going to the bathroom, writing something down, and taking a drink of water. Also correct. In fact, most actions fall into the category of task completion. Whether it occurs under the extreme circumstances of an emergency situation or it is an innocuous task like taking a drink, we spontaneously organize our anatomy to get it done. Task completion just means moving on autopilot.

Check the Rig

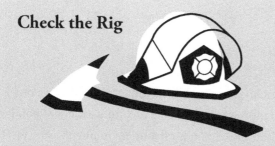

When I was first developing the curriculum for my Check Engine Light class, I bounced some of the core concepts off of my friend and veteran New York City firefighter Felix Manjarrez. In addition to his regular duties, Felix is an FDNY health and fitness unit instructor and a training coordinator in the Office of Professional Development. We were discussing the standard operating procedures for caring for the many pieces of equipment that firefighters use in the course of their job—helmet, flashlight, portable radio, hand tools, and so on. This gear check, or "checking the rig," ensures that things work how they must, when they must. What I found interesting is that the firefighters check their gear *every day* but have no system in place for checking in with their own bodies—a fact that Felix and others in the department are working to change. Like most of us, these firefighters have an implicit assumption that their bodies will just work how they think they should. Until they don't.

When I talk to tactical professionals about task completion, it means to them the kind of attitude that helps firefighters save lives or assists law enforcement officers in catching criminals. The task completion attitude for these folks is to get it done at all costs because they must—it's the kind of thinking that completes missions when things are at their most difficult. This mindset is a beautiful one under the right circumstances, and because of it, people in these professions surmount unbelievable obstacles and at times perform near-miracles. But sometimes it comes back to haunt them, especially when it comes to the care of their own frame.

Always Adapting

The human movement system is a complex, continual, and adaptive orchestration of tension, angles, and vectors that serve to automatically respond to how you orient yourself to the demands of your environment. The vast majority of the time, you simply allow your interaction with the environment to dictate how you move without any explicit standard of execution. This strategy is effective 99.99 percent of the time. It's important to remember, however, that as adaptive as the human body is, its primary modus operandi is not to maintain optimized function in your joints throughout your seventies and eighties. It simply adapts to the inputs that are placed on it, whether you are a conscious participant in that process or not.

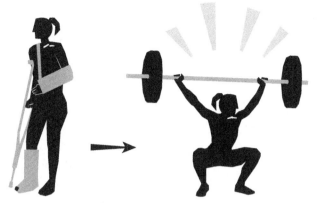

The accumulation of those inputs, whether by conscious selection, training, trauma, or plain ol' repetition of life, have an effect on the way we move. On the whole, this is a good thing. It's a part of what makes us so adaptable. My wife, Thomi, broke her collarbone in a motorcycle accident when she was sixteen. It was not properly set, and as a result, her collarbone on that side looks like two overlapping index fingers. When she raises her hands over her head, one arm is significantly functionally "shorter" than the other. But guess what? She can still reach her arms overhead as well as perform pull-ups, push-ups, and even some Olympic-style weightlifting maneuvers. But it's not as though the adaptation that took place comes with no cost. When Thomi does certain exercises, the injured side gets more sore. The muscles around her neck and shoulder blade on that side get stiff, and that sometimes contributes to headaches. What a beautifully adaptive strategy, however imperfect or asymmetrical.

The Upside of Automatic

The upside of automatic is that it saves a ton of cognitive energy. If you've ever recovered from an injury, you know how mentally exhausting it is to be acutely aware of every little action you're engaging in with that part of your body. It becomes a drag to perform simple tasks that you would normally do without a second thought, let alone anything that might demand a higher level of performance from you. The human movement machine is set up such that as many tasks as possible can be oriented into automatic responses so that cognitive resources can be reserved for solving more complex problems. This automaticity can, on one hand, enhance your ability to perform everyday tasks as well as perform in more demanding environments like sports or emergency situations. In those cases, you want your body to simply do what it was trained to do, whether it's tying your shoes quickly to get out the door on time for work or executing the perfect move to win a game.

The capacity to effectively tune in to the greater problem(s) that need to be solved and tune out the nuanced cognitive burden of conscious body motion is an inherent biological design. But when there is a failure to tap into a deeper awareness, the compensatory abilities embedded in the realm of task completion can create bigger issues down the line. Even if there aren't any easily discernible problems, being stuck in a task completion mindset can send you on a path of adaptation that you aren't even aware of. Many athletes I have worked with over the years had made no connection between subtleties in their movement behavior and outcomes they were getting in training or on the field of play. That may seem somewhat counterintuitive, but athletes often perform well in spite of poor range of motion and movement quality. That's not the issue at hand, though. The issue is, is just doing it enough to sustain health and performance on the long road? My experience working with everyone from everyday people to those at the highest levels of performance says no.

It's kind of like driving around with your tires a little out of balance. Maybe you notice when it first starts to pull, but after a while, you get accustomed to holding the wheel a bit to the side. If you ignore things long enough, you can end up with junky steering, bad shocks, and, if you're really lucky, a brand-new suspension. The problems build and build until a small thing turns into a big issue that "came out of nowhere." (If I had a nickel for every time an athlete said that to me....) This is because humans are master compensators. The same adaptive strategies that welded the broken pieces of my wife's collarbone back together can also create blind spots that build up under the radar. While it makes sense that the most basic software runs on autopilot, it's not enough if you are committed to

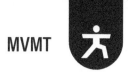

squeezing the most juice out of life. Just like we discussed in the previous chapter on MIND, you need reliable indicators that give you important information so you can regularly audit your ability to move. That's why you need formal movement practices.

SELF-REFLECTION QUESTIONS

Is there a time when having a task completion attitude about MVMT went too far for you? (For example, you were on autopilot and your body built a movement habit or compensation that took away from your ability to move well long term.)

In retrospect, were there any leading indicators that were trying to warn you? Do you have leading indicators in the form of formal movements that you use on a regular basis?

What exercises do you use to gain insight into how well your body is moving?

Formal Movement

Things that take place in a formal environment require adherence to some degree of standards. A formal gala, for example, requires a certain standard of attire and behavior. Formal movement is movement in which you pay strict attention to how you are moving according to a standard of motion. As I'll discuss in the coming sections, the standards of human movement are under constant arbitration among experts. What matters most is that you develop some metric of how *your* body should be able to move and that you have a valid, reliable, and accessible set of KPIs that let you know whether or not you need maintenance.

Formal movement standards can be expressed in biomechanical terms that describe joint kinematics (the way joint surfaces align and interact to produce larger movements), motor control, and tissue quality, all of which add up to produce mathematically definable values for human motion. But let's face it, most movement professionals don't know that stuff. So, while it can be helpful information at the highest levels of precision, very often more easily applied surrogates are sufficient to get the outcome we want: moving better.

I coached CrossFit from around 2007 until Thomi and I closed our gym, CrossFit Virginia Beach, in 2020. CrossFit is a system of fitness that relies on various barbell, calisthenic, and cardiovascular training to elicit a strong exercise stimulus. There always have been and always will be mixed opinions about CrossFit and its use as an exercise modality. I can for sure say that I am thankful for two things about that time in my career: First, I learned how to maintain the attention of a group of adult learners. Working with adults makes you cut out the fluff and get to the point. After a long day of work and paying hard-earned money, people want the goods. Second, I got an ungodly number of repetitions watching human beings move under stress—the truth serum of human motion. This was immensely helpful to me in learning to recognize movement patterns and even predict compensations.

Coinciding with my time as a coach on the training floor was my job as a manual therapist. Using various hands-on massage, neuromuscular, and stretching techniques, I helped clients who were recovering from injury, dealing with chronic pain, and restoring efficient movement patterns. This provided insight into the micro view of movement. I could literally feel with my own two hands how local areas of tissue had responded to the terrain of this person's life. It's the combined lessons I learned from these experiences that highlight the points that follow.

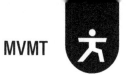

I Was Blind

During my time working as a massage therapist and a coach working with athletes, I learned something that surprises lots of people: Good athletes don't necessarily have any better sense of their movement, in terms of formal and normative value, than the rest of us. They usually have a better sense of performance outcomes and how to achieve them, but not necessarily a better understanding of what is going on under the hood. On one hand, they need to be able to focus on external outcomes and allow their bodies to self-organize to spontaneously solve problems that arise. That's part of what makes good athletes good. The other side of that double-edged blade is that the best athletes are also very often the best compensators. Their bodies will contort and adapt so that the job gets done. Which is all fine and dandy, until it isn't. Then small issues build up, performance takes a hit, and maybe even an injury occurs.

All too often, athletes who would land in my office were painfully unaware of just how far they'd strayed from basic movement standards until it presented a problem. During our assessments, I would use movement tests (some of which I'll discuss in more detail later in this chapter) both in the gym and on the treatment table to break the athletes away from a task completion mindset. These formal movement assessments have demonstrable standards that helped provide a benchmark in both movement quality and quantity so that they could develop a better sense of both how they ended up where they were and how to measure their movement progress into the future.

Whether you are an Olympian or a weekend pickleball devotee, you have little compensations, insults, and adaptations that have built up over time. This unique collection of peccadilloes are what constitute your personal movement signature. Even though there are some clear biomechanical invariants for human motion, within that range is wiggle room for personal expression based on genetics and movement history. That means that on the whole, there are normative measurable ranges of motion, but there is no such thing as "perfect" movement. There are only *stable* patterns of movement.

Let me offer a personal anecdote to illustrate exactly what I mean.

I've dislocated my right shoulder at least four times. The first two were in judo as a young kid. (It's super fun to cry in front of all of your peers at judo camp and then again at a tournament a couple months later, in case you were wondering.) The third time I was body surfing in shore break and got tossed onto the sand. I tried to plant my hand hard as a natural reflex. That one hurt me badly enough that I couldn't slide the back glass closed in my pickup truck with my right hand for three or four months. The last one occurred when I was trying to save a failed attempt at a 300-pound overhead squat. Instead of just ditching the bar, I tried to pull it back into place. Dumb. No pressing overhead for a year.

This series of injuries over the years has resulted in some noticeable differences between my two shoulders. Day to day, they both function normally and without pain, but my right rotator cuff fatigues more quickly and, according to formal, normative values, is less mobile than my left. I work to keep it healthy, but because of the injuries I've sustained, it's just different. However, not only do I know that my right shoulder is further from the ideal in general, but I also know *my own stable ranges of movement quantity and quality within normative ranges.*

To summarize that point, it's important to have some sense of the standard or ideal, where your own values fall in regard to that ideal, and if that is acceptable to you or if it's contributing to problems you might be having.

If you have a way to standardize and become more deeply aware of your movement, you are less likely to get caught off guard by problems in the future. This is true whether you are a high-performing athlete or somebody who just wants to sustain a higher quality of life. Later in this chapter, I'll go deeper into how to develop formal approaches to movement that can help you foster awareness of your body as well as tools that you can deploy to move the needle in the right direction.

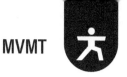

But Now I See

Most of us get out of bed, drink coffee, drive to work (seated), work (often seated), drive home, eat, and then get into bed. That represents the full continuum of the motion of our bodies for the day. Our homogeneous modern environment affords us the opportunity to largely ignore the need for broad movement capacity—that is, until fate thrusts the circumstance upon us where these capacities are required. It's easy to fall prey to the illusion that the bland post-industrial-era, civil-engineered environment of flat sidewalks, escalators, and perfectly squared stairs shows us. Because we are no longer required to use a wide variety of motions to navigate our environment, even the fittest among us become stale and sterilized to the fundamental needs of motion.

Picture a group of typical Westerners on a hike in even mildly challenging terrain. It's not just cardiovascular fitness that can limit participation; it is the inability to tackle simple problems like balancing on a log to cross a small, shallow creek. This is not hypothetical. I've seen it with my own eyes under very mild conditions. Even if you have no plans for outdoor water crossings in the near future, you will, at some point, find yourself in a situation where your lack of movement capacity may surprise you. While no one can be equipped for every possible endeavor, knowing where you stand is a good place to start if you want to be better prepared for the surprises life tends to throw our way.

In Chapter 3, I mentioned my good friend Mickey Schuch, personal defense instructor extraordinaire. Mick hosts a yearly event called the S12 Challenge where interdisciplinary instructors gather in rural Tennessee to instruct civilian students in Stop the Bleed first-aid training as well as basic self-defense and firearms training all with the mission "To Live a Long Full Life" and be of service to your family and your community. While this event is a life-changing experience all around, one of the biggest and often unexpected "aha moments" for many of the participants is realizing how lackluster their ability to move their body has become.

We perform movement drills each morning that require us to skillfully get up and down off the ground in preparation for the more advanced training that occurs later in the day. The amount of groaning, gasping, and overall displeasure that accompanies the reports of surprise is nothing short of astounding. One common comment is, "I didn't even know I couldn't do that because I just don't get exposed to it." In the context of this particular event, self-protection, what happens if you fall or get knocked down in an emergency? How helpful can you be to another person if you can't even get your own carcass off the ground? The point here isn't to beat people over the head with fitness shaming. The point is that most of these people are willing to do something to fix this issue once they know it exists. But they hadn't previously been required to perform to any standard of motion that would clearly expose these deficiencies. That's what formal movement is for.

Formal movement practices offer you a systematic way to establish baseline standards for both the quality and the quantity of your movement capabilities. You can establish a communication rhythm with your muscles and joints so you can be more attuned to the needs of your body. Otherwise, noisy signals like pain and compensation are the sole sources of information for how you're doing.

While the drills we use for this purpose at S12 may be somewhat novel, the concept of needing a formal dialogue with the body is as old as humankind. Ancient spiritual and warrior traditions are rife with systems of physical exploration. Eastern practices like tai chi and yoga are so old it is almost impossible to properly age them. Regardless of their modern iterations, practices like these originally offered the user a series of postures and motions that provided feedback for how well the tires were spinning and an easy route to begin balancing them. Lessons from these ancient movement systems combined with a modern scientific understanding of human motion can give us access to simple and robust practices that you can use to take better stock and care of your frame, regardless of where you're starting from.

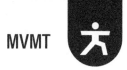

Do you have a formal movement practice in place? How does it inform your choices about how you use your body?

If not, how can you start doing function checks for your body? Name two or three examples of basic movements you are going to do every day for this purpose. Use examples from this book or come up with your own.

Of the examples of formal movement traditions that have been presented, which one resonates most with you and why?

DEVELOPING AWARENESS: INDICATORS FOR MVMT

Getting more attuned to your movement capacity requires you to have measurements you can trust to give you valid and reliable information about your body. Those metrics can come in the form of high-precision technologies that attach numerical value to movement, or they can be a bit more intuitive and holistic in nature. The types you tend to choose probably have as much to do with personal preference as they do with the precision of their outcomes. In my experience, if you're a professional in the movement space, you probably need a good understanding of both, but if you're a person who just wants to feel better, knowing how many degrees of internal rotation your femur requires in extension isn't a must. With that said, let's take a look at some indicators from each category as a way to improve your understanding of the big picture.

Degrees of Freedom: Movement Math

Kinesiology and biomechanics are the study and description of human movement in space, respectively. These fields use physics to observe and explain how a person moves according to established values of joints and muscles and then create a plan for improving the identified patterns of motion. In athletic and surgical settings, tools like goniometers (a sort of protractor for people used in measuring joint angles), motion-tracking cameras and software, and special tests for indicating movement quantity and quality are often used in conjunction to help practitioners better articulate problems and goals in human movement. This makes it easier to set up KPIs so you can measure what can be improved.

There are literally hundreds of tests that kinesiologists use to get information about movement of the body, but let's focus on a few examples that you can try to get some insight into your movement potential. The tests that are employed in physical therapy and sports medicine settings are very granular indicators of movement. In my experience, they are not particularly meaningful to individuals not in those professions and often fail to connect people to something they understand. With that said, I'm going to show a couple of examples just to illustrate the point of how precise normative values can be.

Special Test 1: Shoulder Flexion

This is a test for flexion of the shoulder joint. The head of the humerus (upper arm bone) sits in the socket (glenoid). This test uses specific standards to emphasize the motion of the shoulder complex as the arm is raised overhead. According to the American Academy of Orthopedic Surgeons, normative shoulder flexion is 180 degrees on average.

Perform the test to the following standards:

1. Sit or stand with your upper body and head pressed up against a wall.

2. Engage your abdominals.

3. Lock your elbow straight with the palm of the tested arm facing forward at your side.

4. Keep your arm straight as you raise it overhead.

Avoid:

- Flaring your ribs

- Bending your elbow

- Pushing your head forward

180°

0°

Your measurable range of shoulder flexion is how far you can raise your arm overhead while maintaining the standards described. These standards allow for highly valid and reliable comparisons for shoulder range of motion.

Special Test 2: Hip Flexion

Hip flexion is the closing of the front angle of the hip joint, which is comprised of the thigh bone (femur) and the front of the pelvis (anterior superior iliac spine). This movement is essential in activities like walking up stairs. The standard for hip flexion according to the American Academy of Orthopedic Surgeons is 120 degrees.

Perform the test to the following standards:

1. Lie flat on the ground with your legs extended and your arms by your sides.

2. Keep your foot and knee in alignment with your hip for the entirety of the test.

3. Press the leg you will not be bending into the ground.

4. Keep the toes of both feet actively pointed toward the ceiling.

5. Without assistance from your hands, pull your knee in a straight line toward your torso, bending at the hip and knee.

Avoid:

- Allowing your knee to fall to the inside or outside of your hip line

- Allowing your foot to swing to the inside or outside of the line of your hip

- Allowing your other leg to rise off the floor at all

Your range of hip flexion is measured by the angle between your torso and femur. This test is a valid and reliable indicator for hip flexion range of motion.

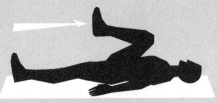

The Bigger Picture: Comprehensive Indicators

You may have noticed that I used two common words to describe indicators: valid and reliable. But what about accessible? There are many, many more special tests like for range of motion and others for additional aspects of total kinesthesia. They're used in physical therapy and sports performance clinics the world over. In this day and age, you can even download apps that will use your phone's camera to assess your range of motion and suggest exercises for you to do. Precision has its place, that's for sure. Especially for medical practitioners. How can we take the same commitment to standards and make it more palatable and accessible so that we all can benefit from increased movement awareness? Let's take a peek at a couple of examples of more comprehensive and accessible benchmarks for movement. I'll use two comprehensive indicators—the overhead press and the squat—as corollary indicators for shoulder flexion and hip flexion, respectively.

Overhead Pressing

Overhead pressing implements of various sorts, used in various ways, has long been a test of upper body strength. More than that, pressing overhead can be a window into overall shoulder function. Pressing any implement overhead is by definition ending in shoulder flexion, as are common bodyweight positions like handstands, downward-facing dog in yoga, and hanging from a pull-up bar.

Bringing your arms overhead is an easy range of motion to take for granted—until you lose it. Awareness and development of overhead pressing may not seem like a necessary part of your repertoire, especially if you're not at athlete. However, including it can be a wonderful litmus test for shoulder health in general and can contribute to the maintenance of a wider menu of movement options to navigate the world.

Getting reliable information means you need a standard of execution. Let's take a look standards for the overhead press.

Note: There may be some minor differences depending on the implement being pressed, but the majority of the standards will hold true regardless.

- Stand with your feet, knees, hips, shoulders, and head stacked in alignment.

- Create tension in your lower body and torso.

- Balance the implement of choice on your shoulder(s) and over your feet.

- Push the implement straight up.

- Stop when the implement is over your head.

- The ideal finish position is when your body is in alignment with the implement over your head, your elbows locked, and your biceps pointing toward your ears.

Avoid:

- Bending your elbows

- Bending your knees

- Arching your back or flaring your ribs out

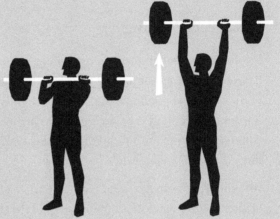

Squatting

Squatting is often thought of as an exercise to build leg strength, which it is, but fundamentally it is a position for resting and defecation. The ability to sit down relaxed in the bottom of a squat to rest or poop is, in terms of global movement behavior, the norm in the world to this day. I affectionately refer to this kind of squat as the mahjong squat because years ago I saw a picture of a bunch of old Chinese men with long white beards who were playing mahjong on a street corner while smoking cigarettes. Every single one was chillin' out in the bottom of a squat.

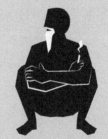

Performing a squat is a quite literally the ability to stay balanced on two feet while your lower your torso by bending your ankles, knees, and hips. Effectively, this is flexion of all three of those joint spaces at once. Let's examine the squat a bit more closely.

Perform the test to the following standards:

- Stand upright with your feet somewhere between hip and shoulder width apart.

- Point your feet somewhere between straight ahead and 20 degrees outward.

- Keep both feet flat with pressure in the three points of the foot (big toe, little toe, and heel) throughout the movement.

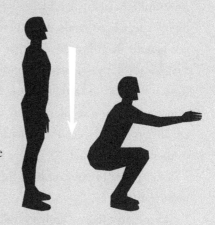

- Inhale and descend by bending at the ankle, knee, and hip.

- Keep your torso as upright as possible the entire time.

- You've reached the bottom when you get as low as possible while maintaining the above conditions.

- Press your feet into the ground to stand up.

- Perform 3 to 5 times to get a good read.

Avoid:

- Lifting your heels

- Lifting your toes

- Rounding your back

(These things are not "wrong." They just aren't the standard we are using.)

Sometimes there's pushback on indicators like this from people who use outliers to rationalize their crappy range of motion. Do NBA players need to be able to squat butt to calves in order to be healthy? Can they? The answer to both is probably. They are genetic outliers who have made a conscious choice to specialize in an activity with an extraordinarily high return on investment. I guess what I'm saying is that being a seven-foot-tall multimillionaire freak athlete buys you some wiggle room. If you're not a highly specialized freak, you'd better get those joints flowing. But everyone can benefit from litmus tests that are designed to measure where they stand against normative values and, more importantly, where their movement capacity is relative to their peers. Regardless of whether you're a professional athlete or a regular ol' guy or gal just trying to hold it together, there are always three layers of comparison: 1) Where is your indicator compared to the human normal? 2) Where is it compared to your peers? 3) Where is it compared to yourself over time? (Hint: The third one is the most important one.)

Think of it like an archery bullseye. The X in the center of the target represents a perfect shot. The ideal. Then there is a series of concentric rings that represent getting farther away from the intended target. If you don't hit the bullseye but your arrows are closer together (a tight group), you're in a stable pattern but not quite hitting the target. You're consistent but not quite there. Easy to adjust. If you get an arrow in the 10 ring (the one that encircles the bullseye) but the next three are all over the place, your pattern isn't stable yet. The X in this analogy is the normative movement standards. People don't hit those perfectly very often. But when you move, are your "shots" close together, or are they all over the place? Are you getting closer to the X with more frequency? Do you know what adjustments to make to get closer? Are you trying anything to change where your shots hit? Here's the real clincher—when it comes to how their bodies move, most people don't even have an X that they are aiming at. They're just slinging arrows with fingers crossed that things will work out.

Let's zoom back out for a moment. When it comes to the variety of indicators that are available to standardize human movement, there is an endless supply of both the granular and biomechanical and the more comprehensive. In the world of human movement education and rehabilitation, these standards and how well any given exercise reflects them are under constant arbitration. If you're a person who tends to get a little stuck in the details, I implore you, don't. The examples I have provided are simply to illustrate the point that it's important to have some standardization of movement execution if we want fair comparisons between them. They by no means even remotely represent the vast complexity of what it is to be a human moving. Over time, what matters most is that you have reliable ways to pay attention to your movement health, measure it, and make changes if and when you decide to.

To add to this point, I really do not care if you use the particular metrics I've outlined here or if you agree with the standards. Both are under constant arbitration. Start with these if you don't know of any. But over time, I hope you will learn more and develop your own set of movement indicators. You do this by engaging in regular movement practices as well as pursuing a deeper understanding of the care of your own frame.

MVMT Feel: Beyond Mathematics

It is important to have standardized values of your own motion so you can generate comparisons over time. But equally important is your felt experience of how your body moves. After all, you don't experience 180 degrees of shoulder flexion; you experience how your shoulder feels when you raise your arm over your head. Standardized ranges, such as the examples we explored in the previous section, should work in tandem with your internal movement sense. Remember, they serve to calibrate your perception and hone your kinesthetic awareness. Use them, but be sure they serve you, not the other way around.

As you work at improving the performance longevity of your movement, you might not notice a measurable change in range of motion per se, but instead an improvement in the quality of your movement experience. By mathematical improvement standards, that's not moving the needle in the right direction, strictly speaking, but you experience your body through your senses, not through rulers. Measuring movement is important, but equally important is developing a better sense of feel. But how can we measure the subjective intangible? It is certainly difficult, but one way is through self-reflection using mood words. Mood words summarize internal feeling states. Coaches and athletes often use mood words to summarize the intentions behind movements in practice and competition.

Mood words evoke an emotional response or feeling. When you apply mood words to movement, they can help you summarize a feeling or intention. It can be difficult to determine what delineates "good" human movement from "bad," especially when there isn't a change in a strictly measurable outcome. With that said, somehow we can sense quality movement when we see it or feel it, especially if we purposefully develop our ability to do so over time.

One group of people who work diligently to develop their sense of movement are professional coaches. Not only do coaches need a fundamental understanding of biomechanics and quantities of athlete motion, but they also need to possess the ability to describe the quality of motion. Savvy communication using mood words can be used to succinctly describe the quality of an exercise to an athlete or cue the athlete to change their behavior quickly. Mood words in athletic performance speak to the feeling behind movements and allow athletes to label the internal summary of how a movement feels. My good friend Stu MacMillan of ALTIS uses words like *glide, float, grind, steady,* and *persist* as "motor shortcuts" to cut out technical jargon and more efficiently elicit changes in his athletes' movement behavior. Mood words can also help you improve your internal dialogue and self-reflection so that you can develop a more sophisticated dialogue with your own body.

These types of intuitive indicators don't have to be limited to athletes, either. You can use mood words to amplify your internal dialogue about your own movement. In my experience, tuning in to movement moods, if you will, can help excavate a deeper rapport with the sensations of your own body.

To further illustrate this idea, I asked more than a dozen coaches in my contact list what mood words they use to describe athlete movement. I prompted the coaches I polled to provide three to five words that describe "good" movement versus "bad" movement from their subjective point of view. Certainly, the array of what constitutes human movement is vastly more complex than "good" versus "bad," but it's a good place to start the conversation. Check out the list to see how the coaches responded.

GOOD	BAD
Efficient, clean, controlled, precise	Inefficient, chaotic, imprecise, sloppy
Sharp, strong, smooth, aware, efficient	Dull, weak, inefficient
Rhythmic, graceful, balanced, relaxed	Rigid, clumsy, jerky, tense
Connected, fluid, organized, pristine, polished	Erratic, disoriented, incomplete, sloppy, brittle
Fluid, pretty, smooth, natural	Junky, rigid, uncontrolled, disconnected
Crisp, fluid, deliberate, nimble, swift	Loose, cumbersome, dopey, sloppy
Bouncy, focused, powerful, vigorous, quick	Slow, frail, feeble, chaotic, stiff
Steady, deliberate, controlled	Inconsistent, sporadic, lacking
Fluid, effortless, strategic	Hesitant, forced
Controlled, precise	Erratic, weird, anxious, ditzy
Bouncy, relaxed, powerful	Sluggish, rigid, hunched
Heavy, tall, striding	Slow, rigid, hesitant, sloppy, rushed
Fluid, connected, smooth	Stiff, chaotic, choppy
Agile, punchy, flexible	Awkward, clunky, bumpy

You might have noticed that there are some repeat offenders on this list of mood words. *Fluid, smooth,* and *controlled* topped the list for good movement. Alongside those, descriptors like efficient and powerful were also used. On the side of bad movement quality, *rigid* and *sloppy* topped out. Mood words like these can be personal to the coach and to the athlete. Some of them will probably speak to you, and others won't. I recommend zoning in on the ones that conjure up a feeling in your own bodily experience and using them as a tool for calibrating your own movement.

Can You Try New Things?

The greatest sign of movement literacy and longevity isn't necessarily being good at things in the narrow groove you've worn into your nervous system, no matter how well you've preserved specific capacities or ranges. It isn't passing a range of motion, balance, or agility test, either. Perhaps the greatest sign is whether or not you can try and learn new things. Think for a moment about people you know who throughout their lives and into advanced age are willing to take risks, to learn new skills, and to play. Those people tend to be full of vitality and zest. The kind of confidence that emerges from possessing an adaptable body that moves well allows you to approach life knowing that you can more readily march toward challenges whether they are thrust upon you or you decide to pursue them to more fully experience joie de vivre. Of course, this capacity takes more work to preserve as you age. But a consistent attitude of playful exploration and thoughtful challenge is a key aspect to preserving movement and helps you maintain a more lucid self-assessment of your faculties.

To that end, go try new things. They don't have to be complete departures from what you are used to. A few degrees from center is a good place to start for most people. Put yourself in an unfamiliar situation or environment that tests you and develops your ability to puzzle out the dark and dusty corners of your body. As a personal example, I like to try out different strength and conditioning programs. I don't jump around picking exercises off a buffet every week. That's a fast track to nowhere. Instead, I'll pick a training program that sounds interesting and commit to it for a minimum of one year. Most recently, it's been a mixture of heavy kettlebell and mace work by Subversive Fitness. I also played handball with my wife for the first time. Both showed me places my movement preservation strategies had succeeded up to that point as well as gaps in my capacity that could be improved upon. You don't necessarily need to do those particular activities, but the larger takeaway is building a strong enough movement vocabulary that you can play on the playground rather than sit on the bench and watch the other kids have fun.

SELF-REFLECTION QUESTIONS

Take a moment to think about what you've learned so far about calibrating perception by using better indicators and tools. Now let's apply those same concepts to the category of MVMT.

Can you think of a situation in which you ignored indicators related to MVMT? Describe it here.

Were you unaware of the indicator, did you interpret it incorrectly, or did you just ignore it?

What happened as a result?

I LIKE TO MOVE IT: TOOLS FOR IMPROVING MVMT

It's one thing to become more aware of your movement. It's another thing to know how to go about maintaining or improving. To start, I'll discuss some general ideas to improve your range of motion and movement quality. Please keep in mind that the options presented here are not the everything of moving better. As a rule, I'm agnostic, with the caveat that there has to be some demonstrable outcome in the thing you are trying to change. Let's start with the most obvious.

Just Move

Before you go getting all fancy with mystical movement techniques, the first thing you can do if you want to preserve movement is—drumroll, please—move. Find opportunities in your day to get up and move around. Pursue a variety of hobbies that expose you to different ways of moving, or pursue a single hobby that requires a variety of movement, like dance classes or martial arts. Getting outside to walk or hike in different environments can expose you to novel movement challenges. Natural environments in particular are usually full of fun surprises that challenge problem solving in both mind and body.

A few years back, after an uncharacteristic snowfall in Virginia Beach, I went on a hike with my wife and some friends. Marsh streams were flowing way higher than normal. We had to balance on fallen logs that had patches of ice, jump over creeks, and sidewind up frozen sand dunes. All fun and interesting ways to explore and build our movement repertoire. If you happen to be in a more urban environment, there are still plenty of ways to keep your body moving in weird and wonderful ways. While you may not go full-throttle into parkour, even simple things like taking the stairs two or three at a time are subtle probes into your movement.

Less broadly speaking, if you want to improve your ability to perform a specific movement, the easiest thing is to practice that movement. For example, earlier in this chapter, we examined overhead pressing and squats

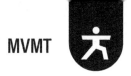
as types of movement indicators. One of the simplest things you can do to improve those movements and subsequently the ranges of motion they express is to regularly perform them to the given standard—that is, executing exercises using full range of motion.

The next question you might ask is, how often? In response to your question, I offer another: How important is it to you? When I coached people in these movements and we found a problem they were committed to change, we would make it a part of their training routine every day.

Whether it's a specific range of motion or the maintenance of movement intelligence overall, movement practices that offer both the opportunity to practice to a standard and also develop a wide array of capacities is a good way to go.

Stretching

If I'm being totally honest, a part of me is hesitant to write this section. First, stretching is a pretty ambiguous term. In the marketplace of feel-good bodies, not all tools are created equal but may share the same categorization. Second, its effect on performance, at least according to recent research, is unclear. What is clear, however, both in terms of research and my own practical experience, is that stretching tools, when used thoughtfully, can be pathways to a deeper connection with your body and create space and comfort in local areas that can provide access to new movement possibilities. Then you can do the thing that is guaranteed to grant you better movement: movement itself.

When you think of stretching, you might think of pulling the two ends of a rubber band apart to increase the length of the rubber band. Human bodies don't quite work like that. Our movement machines are complex systems of bones, joints, muscles, nerves, and connective tissues, each with a distinct contribution to the net effect of movement. Often, when people stretch, they reach the first barrier to movement, hang out there just long enough to eke out a grimace, and then call it quits. Insufficient doesn't begin to describe how lackluster most efforts to improve range of motion are.

Let's be more specific with the outcome we want, then. We want to improve access to larger ranges of motion. Instead of just pulling the rubber band apart for half a second and expecting change, we need to spend time under tension. The amount of time can vary from short periods such as ten seconds all the way up to two or three minutes spent in one position. What seems to be more important than acute stretch time is collected time in the end range position. One to two minutes collected per position per session seems to be a good place to start.

This basic style of stretching is often referred to as static passive stretching, although that term is a bit of misnomer because when you execute it properly, you're not passive at all. I prefer the more specific term *end range isometrics*. This means taking tissues to their end range of motion and periodically creating tension in the muscles in that limb without moving it. This gets the nervous system involved in an acceptable reset of the movement.

Most improvements in movement, especially in the short term, come from changes in the proprioceptors, the nerves found in the joints, muscles, and tendons. An interesting display of this phenomenon is how flexible patients become when they are under anesthesia. One minute they look like they're made from old gum stuck under a middle school desk, and the next they could try out for the circus. Did their muscles suddenly get longer? No, the tone of their nervous system decreased. With that said, we're not going to get that relaxed no matter what we do, nor do we want to. Some level of tone in the body is necessary to stabilize our movement. The lesson to be learned, however, is that if you want stretching to work, you have get the nervous system involved.

Contract/Relax Stretching

One of the easiest tools to integrate into your own movement practice is contract/relax. Here are the guidelines to get started with an easy example to try:

1. Find your pain-free end range of motion in the movement pattern you want to change.

2. Take a deep breath and hold it.

3. Squeeze the muscles in that part of your body tight for three to five seconds.

4. Exhale slowly as you relax.

5. Explore the position for newly available end range of motion.

6. Repeat three to five times for one to two minutes.

Feel free to combine this tool with more dynamic movement that uses this end range of motion.

One of the cool side benefits of using a tool like contract/relax stretching is that it not only is a way to involve the nervous system but also provides another layer of insight into the mood of your nervous system from day to day. One thing we look for in the therapeutic environment is how a person's nervous system responds to manual inputs. If, for example, I was deploying this technique on a therapy client, I would be looking for not only a net increase in range of motion but also how well their nervous system responded to the stimulus in general.

How does this help you? Well, imagine you did a series of movements or stretches every morning to start your day. Somewhere in there, you might realize that you're a little stiff and do a little contract/relax to nudge things in the right direction. Now, normally when you do that, you get a nice little bump in your range of motion. But today, you didn't. That doesn't mean the sky is falling, but it does tell you something about the overall condition of your body. Maybe you're feeling the effects of yesterday's hike? Maybe you're dehydrated? Maybe you slept weird? It's hard to know exactly in one isolated situation. But what you do have, and what speaks to the larger overall theme of this book, is a more layered and sophisticated awareness of your movement. More on how to put this all of together later in this chapter.

Stretching exercises have the potential to improve body awareness and range of motion when used with enough frequency and intention. There are a multitude of resources out there that can help you get started. Some of my favorites can be found in the resources section of this book.

FORMAL MVMT SYSTEMS

Range of motion indicators and tools are an important slice of the movement pie, but remember that they don't fill the whole pan. Other qualities like strength, agility, power, coordination, accuracy, and even grace are all gods in the pantheon. Movement religion cannot be monotheistic. All of the parts come together to congeal into human movement. While basic movements like overhead pressing and bodyweight squats may not be all that and a bag of chips in terms of sophistication, they and indicators like them are great starting places for creating standard values in quantity and quality of movement. These data points can then be tracked over time and context. All to enhance attunement with your own body.

Back when I was coaching CrossFit with my wife, Thomi, I noticed that one of the hidden benefits of CrossFit is that it can provide insight to participants about how their bodies move. The pop culture representation of that environment is mostly people flailing around until they're super sweaty and tired with the occasional box jump fall or pull-up catastrophe. If I'm telling the truth, those things do happen in the broader world of CrossFit (never in our gym though, wink). But when executed well, CrossFit provides an opportunity to engage in a practice that can define normative ranges of motion for people in a way that makes sense and can be practically applied.

That is actually a major purpose of exercise and strength and conditioning environments in general: to supply the "athlete" with a formal language of movement attributes so that they, alongside their coaches, can identify and alleviate weak links in their overall capacity. Using the physical training

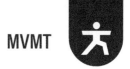

and exercise environments in this way is, in my experience, also one of the biggest lost opportunities in all of human performance.

How can you engage with formal movement practice if you're not into CrossFit or don't have access to high-level performance environment? You can start by paying closer attention to what you're already doing. Then you can learn good form for those exercises from a valid and reliable resource so that you can produce consistent movement patterns to a standard over time. Your understanding of that form will most certainly evolve, but what matters most is that you have a standard to begin with.

Not only can formal standards of movement be integrated into an existing exercise program by understanding how to perform exercises with proper range of motion, but they can also be separate practices unto themselves that further develop your awareness without the chance to get unwillingly drawn back into task completion modes of operation. Some of these systematized movement practices have been a part of human culture for thousands of years with the exact purpose of harmonizing awareness of mind and body.

The Best of the Best and All the Rest

ALTIS is one of the premiere training groups in the world for track and field. Collegiate, professional, and Olympic athletes pick up their lives and move to Phoenix, Arizona, to train with the elite staff of coaches and therapists who call ALTIS home. ALTIS is known throughout the sports performance world as the place to be not only if you want to be the best of the best in your sport, but also if you want to be the best of the best in coaching.

The ALTIS team has spent decades studying the movement of athletes, systematizing and cataloging various patterns and shapes and from that creating a language that can be used to describe the formal movements of sports, sprinting in particular. Kinograms, originally developed by CEO Stu MacMillan and head coach Dan Pfaff, are freeze-frame images that help athletes and coaches more accurately capture and analyze key movement signatures in the cycle of sprinting. Based on these standards of motion, coaches can offer cues, recommendations, and interventions to help athletes move and perform more effectively.

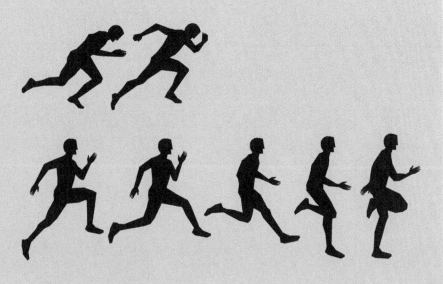

Recording these kinograms has two important effects. First, it helps coaches and athletes compare their normal movement signature to the standard for performance across all athletes. These normative values provide a baseline for how most elite sprinters solve the same movement problems. In fact, establishing normative values for motion is an important part of what formal movement practices do for all of us. Additionally, it helps tune coaches' eyes to important checkpoints in an athlete's movement patterns. This way, they can more clearly monitor consistency in the athlete's patterns as they fatigue during a session and how they react to training and competition stress over time. A sense of what is normal for that individual can also be established, and if their movement starts to veer too far outside of their normal bandwidth, attention can be called to this trend (!) for further investigation before they stray too far and create a pattern that gets more expensive down the line.

So what about the rest of us? Do we need to use the methods of elite athletes to track our movement from day to day in an effort to eke out as much performance as possible? No. And yes. Maybe we don't need a team of coaches standing by performing movement analysis, but we do need a known standard for our range of motions and capacities that we can measure ourselves against over time. Even the simplest standards can have incredibly positive effects. These standards provide consistent feedback that can keep us in the loop so we can see problems coming down the road (leading indicators, again) and course-correct so that things don't get worse than they need to be.

FORMAL MOVEMENT MARKET

The idea of having standards for human motion is not original to this book. Not by a long shot. Taking a look at some historical examples can be helpful as you decide what kinds of movement indicators you might want to place on your Performance Longevity Dashboard. Regardless, if you like one of these formal movement systems more than the others, or none of them at all, the point remains the same—having a standard is necessary lest you be lost in the abyss of waiting until things break.

Feldenkrais Method

Moshe Feldenkrais, a legend among those who work in movement education of any sort, was a Ukrainian-Israeli physicist and engineer. He was an influential and prolific figure. In addition to working on various engineering projects in France, the United Kingdom, and Israel, he played soccer and practiced martial arts, including judo and jiu-jitsu, and wrote multiple books on human movement, philosophy, and martial arts.

A debilitating knee injury from soccer pushed Feldenkrais to use his knowledge of physics and human movement to create Awareness Through Movement, a system of exercises, along with a book of the same name, to increase bodily awareness and actualize human potential. This system utilizes a combination of floor, balance, and postural exercises combined with breathing to initiate a deeper sense of body awareness, or, as practitioners of this method refer to it, somatic connection.

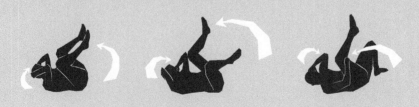

Pilates

Joseph Pilates was a German-American exercise instructor and the inventor of a method of health and fitness that bears his name. Pilates exercises were made famous after being adopted by New York City dance companies in the 1930s, but Joseph Pilates conceived of them during his time in a World War I internment camp in Lancaster Castle, Great Britain.

Although Pilates was a sickly child, his diligent practice of gymnastics and weightlifting turned his health around by his early teens. He used this experience and his later experience as a boxer and gymnast to help his fellow prisoners and soldiers stay healthy during their time together at Lancaster.

Pilates went on to systematize his approach to movement and called it "Contrology," focusing on deep awareness of breath and postural muscles as well as core strength through the use of floor exercises and specially designed machines that he invented. When he emigrated to the United States in the 1920s, he brought his method with him, and it was quickly adopted by professional dancers as a way to prevent and rehabilitate injury.

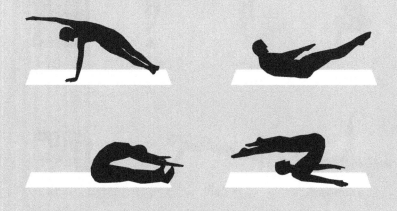

Functional Movement Screen

Gray Cook, MSPT, is the founder of Functional Movement Systems and inventor of the Functional Movement Screen (FMS). The FMS is taught as a standard of care throughout the physical therapy and sports performance world.

The FMS is a series of seven key patterns that offer physical therapists and trainers an objective assessment of a person's movement. Each baseline movement is categorized as optimal, acceptable, or dysfunctional, and the ratings can be used to guide rehabilitative and training programs. These patterns are designed not only to serve as objective metrics but to also improve feedback in the body-patient-practitioner triad.

While the FMS is primarily utilized by movement professionals like strength and conditioning coaches and physical therapists, anybody can find them with a basic internet search and use them as a starting point for analyzing their own movement.

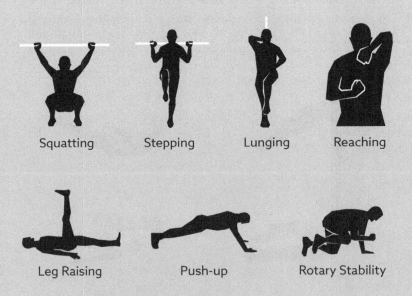

Squatting   Stepping   Lunging   Reaching

Leg Raising   Push-up   Rotary Stability

Becoming a Supple Leopard: The Archetypes

Dr. Kelly Starrett, the author of multiple *New York Times* bestsellers, including his seminal work, *Becoming a Supple Leopard*, has been one of the most prolific figures in the space of performance and pain relief in the last decade. *Becoming a Supple Leopard* offers simple, testable movement standards for the "native" ranges of motion of the human body as well as simple ways to steer the body toward optimal movement expression.

Becoming a Supple Leopard shaped a generation of coaches, physical therapists, and athletes by offering easy-to-understand and apply "archetypes" for human movement based on many of the standard shapes found in strength and conditioning. Along with those archetypal shapes, the book offers simple and easy-to-execute interventions for pain and movement dysfunction using simple and accessible tools.

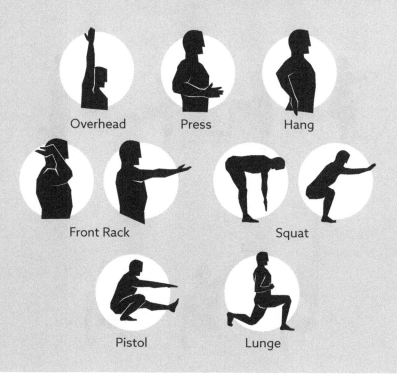

Overhead   Press   Hang

Front Rack   Squat

Pistol   Lunge

Functional Range Systems

Created by world-renowned chiropractor Andreo Spina, Functional Range Systems (FRS) is a coordinated system of manual therapy and movement training that uses specifically designed techniques to "develop mobility, improve joint strength, and increase body control." FRS leans on the scientific research of human movement to develop exercises that improve pain-free motion.

One of the signature components is what Dr. Spina refers to as controlled articular rotations, or CARs. CARs are exercises designed to maintain and improve the functional range of motion of joints through the precise exploration of workspace, the full rotational capacity of a given joint in three-dimensional space. Dr. Spina recommends this series of exercises be performed by his clients "every damn day" in order to maintain the baseline capacity of the specialized mechanical sensors found in our muscles and joints.

Standing Hip CARs

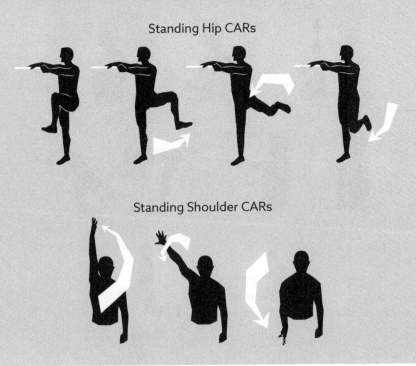

Standing Shoulder CARs

Ido Portal

Ido Portal is probably best known for his work with mixed martial arts legend Conor McGregor. Far more than that, Ido is a teacher and philosopher who has traveled the world many times over teaching students about not just the gross physical aspects of human motion but also the subtle psychological and philosophical lessons that can be learned through the practice of Movement with a capital M.

Two primary human patterns that Ido has expressed as paramount to his view of functional motion are squatting and hanging. His social media squatting and hanging "challenges" invite participants to engage in those respective shapes for a given amount of time each day for thirty days. These challenges attract tens of thousands of participants and offer many a new way to think about the basic functionality of their bodies.

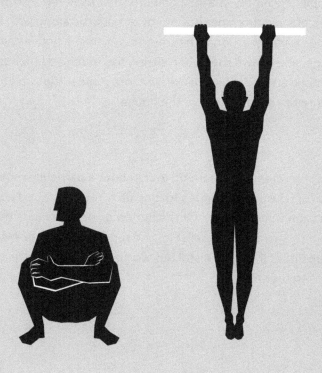

SELF-REFLECTION QUESTIONS

Do you have a formal movement practice in place? How does it inform your choices about how you use your body?

If not, how can you start doing function checks for your body? Name two or three examples of basic movements you are going to do every day for this purpose. Use examples from this book or come up with your own.

Of the examples of formal movement traditions that are presented in this chapter, which one resonates most with you? Why?

Example: My ninety-year-old grandmother uses the trip up the three flights of stairs from her basement to her attic along with her relative perceived exertion as her metric. When she notices a negative change, she knows she's been sitting too much and tries to get up and move around more to include more regular trips up and down the stairs to the second floor of the house.

If you're interested in learning more about a particular movement practice, take a few minutes to look up a YouTube video about exercises from that category. Of the hundreds or thousands that show up, which seem robust, reliable, and repeatable for you? Which ones are proximal? If they're distal but worth the effort, where can you get access to them?

NOTHING NEW

Of course, the idea of standardized movement patterns is nothing new. Martial arts like karate and tae kwon do have included "forms" as part of their practice for centuries. While some good arguments have been made against this practice as an effective means for combat preparation, these series of movements could serve as a way for practitioners to tune into their patterns of movement against a larger standard and to develop a tolerance for motions that may be necessary to train in those martial arts.

Related to these martial practices are practices that could be classified more as moving mediations, like tai chi and yoga. Tai chi, a branch of the tree of Chinese kung fu, is a form of exercise that uses flowing patterns of motion combined with breathing exercises to relax the mind and body and to keep the chi, or vital energy, flowing. Yoga includes both movement (asana) and meditation practices that are also focused on the flow of vital energy through the body to encourage balance and health. Whether or not you believe in any sort of divine vital energy, one thing is for sure: If you want to remain a vital and energetic human being, keeping your body moving is an absolute must.

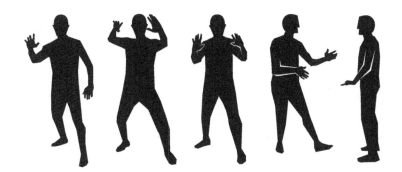

Some of these systems represent more fluid and intuitive approaches, whereas others are more objective and granular. Regardless of which of these particular examples speaks to you (or maybe none of them do), what's truly important is that you have a reliable line of communication with your body about your ability to move through space. You might like a different brand of toothpaste than I do, but the fact remains that we both still need to brush our teeth.

FUNCTION CHECK

When it comes to keeping in tune with whether or not the body is firing on all cylinders, the thing I've relied on most for myself and for my clients over the years is Sun Salutation (Surya Namaskar) from hatha yoga. Sun Salutation is a series of repeating postures that are combined with controlled breathing in a cycle performed at dawn each day as a sort of welcome to the sun, hence the name. This series is often used as a way to introduce beginners to the basic motions of asana (posture) practices. Yogis perform asanas combined with controlled breathing as a way to focus the mind and challenge the body as well as expose any areas that may be limiting their ability to stay focused and relaxed during meditation.

I was introduced to Sun Salutation in college when I took a yoga class at Old Dominion University back in 1999–2000. The instructor, whose name I ashamedly cannot remember, was an excellent teacher from the Iyengar tradition. B. K. S. Iyengar was an instrumental figure in the popularization of yoga exercises in the West and was particularly known for his rigorous approach to proper mechanics in the yoga postures as well as the use of props to help new practitioners appropriately scale their efforts. (Hmm, it's kind of like he was enforcing a normative value of movement through yoga postures...but I digress.) I quickly took to it and have since engaged in a yoga practice that has ranged from deeply obsessed to casual.

As my career and my understanding of a potentially deeper use progressed, my application of this simple series changed. During my time as a massage therapist and later as a coach, I realized that most people need a consistent and easily learnable practice so they can check in on their basic movement capacity from day to day. So I started assigning Sun Salutation to my private clients in the early 2000s and pretty much every client I've worked with since. The results for both my clients and me personally have been nothing short of remarkable. Sun Salutation provides an avenue for dialogue, both internal and external, that can be tracked over time. It also serves as a standard, normative value for some basic and easily understood motions of the human body. When I teach it to military personnel, I liken it to a function check—a simple series of checks performed on a rifle to make sure that it, well, functions. Every grunt learns this procedure in boot camp because not knowing the condition of your weapon prior to needing it in combat could result in death. Makes sense. Why not, then, have a function check for the one tool *every* human being must use to operate in life?

Here's why I've grown to like Sun Salutation so much. First, you can take it anywhere, and it requires little space, little time, and no equipment (Robust). Second, by attending to your breathing (an autonomic nervous system behavior from Chapter 1), you'll get consistent insight into how the deepest layers of your physiology are responding to the movements you're doing (Reliable). Not to mention that it's a nice reboot to the software first thing in the morning. Lastly, as a coach, it's easy for me to teach and easy for my clients to learn and remember (Repeatable). It passes the Mickey Schuch R3 sniff test with a score of 100 percent.

Due to the simplicity of application and the relatively low physical cost, you can do Sun Salutation every single day. That's 365 data points a year that you get from your body about how well you are moving. Over the last twenty-four or so years of using this sequence, I've had the opportunity to develop insight into parts of my health I never would have expected. For instance, I was able to correlate deep sleep data with tightness in my hamstrings and low back. For me, it seems that regardless of any physical input, if I miss out on too much deep sleep, my hips and back feel stiffer.

Sun Salutation in particular may or may not be right for you. I honestly don't know. Regardless of which standard of function you choose, make sure that it is easy for you to use and provides useful information that you understand.

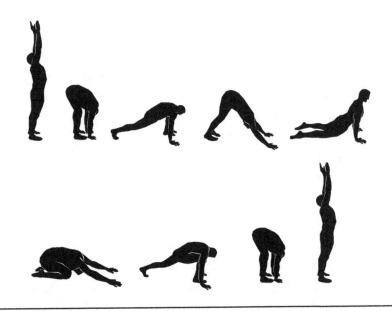

Sun Salutation offers an elegant starting place to tune into the movement of your body. The sequence pictured can be performed as a flow in the order shown or as individual segments. Regardless of which way you do it, remember that the point isn't to perform it to completion but to use each movement as a way to develop a deeper relationship with your body.

DON'T GAME YOUR INDICATORS

A brief word of caution on movement indicators: It's a generally healthy practice to continually audit the purpose any indicator or tool is serving in the context of helping you build performance longevity. It's easy to become attached to indicators, fall prey to biases, and engage in hacks that move the needle on the numbers but may not be relevant to the big picture. I'll use an example from my time as a CrossFit coach.

In the CrossFit methodology, intensity, calculated as work divided by time, is a key feature of progress in general fitness, and as such, there are benchmark workouts designed to test athletes' progress after a period of building fitness. For fun, these workouts are often named. Fran, the Filthy Fifty, and Fight Gone Bad were in the original pantheon of CrossFit tests.

They are most often performed in peer group classes with results publicly displayed and recorded.

On one hand, I think having known and quantifiable benchmarks for testing abilities that you are working to develop is important. "Prove it" isn't just for quelling playground braggadocio. On the other hand, and a serious downside that I saw quite a lot of in the CrossFit gym, is that athletes would lose sight of why they were training in the first place. They looked for ways to hack the system, to specifically improve their scores while neglecting to improve other aspects of their fitness that would serve them over the long haul. They became more "fit" by that standard but were also riddled with -itises and -opathies—all for the pursuit of recreational fitness improvement. As my friend and CrossFit super coach Kenny Kane always says, "Context is king."

When we fixate on Measures of Performance (see Chapter 2), we can become blinded by our pursuit of the A+. We cram for the exam, but we don't learn in ways that are meaningful and lasting. As you pursue both indicators and tools for improving your experience in your body, stay aware of the reason you're doing it in the first place.

RENT'S DUE

Life is full of unavoidable bumps in the road, and the toll that your physical body incurs is no exception to that rule. This book is not about the things that happen to you. Unfortunately, the development of formal movement indicators does not keep you safe from the unpredictable and chaotic world that we live in. In other words, shit happens. Becoming better attuned to the messages that are coming from inside your body is about knowing yourself better, in this case through the vehicle of your own motion.

The point isn't necessarily to replicate any of the specific examples that I have laid out here. The point is to generate a connection between your conscious mind and the state of your body, and to do so in a way that is simple, reliable, and applicable to your circumstances, whatever they may be. It may be through a specific example I provided, or maybe it won't. On television, YouTube, and social media, you'll find a plethora of exercise systems and technologies telling you how to move your body. Everyone tells you that their way is the best and everybody else's stinks. The truth is that much of it works *if you execute it with focus, consistency, and most of all intention.* If that includes one of the practices I talk about in this book, great. If not, that's okay, too. Find something that makes sense to you and commit.

I, for one, am agnostic about it. If doing tai chi keeps you in touch with your body and gets you moving, then tai chi it is. Yoga, StretchLab, Pilates, weightlifting—whatever. My ninety-year-old grandmother uses the stair climb from her basement to her attic as her litmus test of function. If it doesn't harm you and helps you invest in the process of preserving your ability to move well, I'm in. That brings me to my final point: This is a process. Health and performance longevity are not destinations. You don't arrive at health. Health can never be bought; it can only be rented. Movement is no exception.

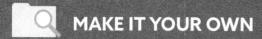 **MAKE IT YOUR OWN**

Deandre Corbe is an engineer by trade but a world-class jiu-jitsu player by craft. He is one of the top-ranked black belts in the world as well as one of the most committed students of health and performance I've ever known.

D and I began working together in an effort to reconfigure his approach to strength and conditioning in preparation for the Pan American and World Championships in the 2019–2020 season. While he was far more attuned than many of the athletes I had worked with in the past, he had not yet developed a formal indicator system that would give him direct and precise insight into his movement quality over time. To fill this gap for the eighteen or so months that D and I worked together, we added Sun Salutation to his prescribed morning ritual.

Deandre eventually moved away, but we've kept in touch. In preparation for writing this chapter, I asked him if he still uses Sun Salutation. His answer: no. However, he has developed his own flow based on other movements he'd tried over time.

Herein lies the truly important point that is easily lost as we collect movement indicators: It is ultimately up to us to take ownership over our own process. Outsourcing is okay, especially when you are first getting started. But you need to make these practices your own and continually upgrade the indicators you put on your dashboard and the tools you put in your toolbox. I'm happy to provide starting places, whether directly to a client or in a book like this one, but the end goal is not rote repetition because somebody says so. It's to make it work for you in your own life—and that is something only you can do.

CHAPTER 6: | MTTR

The third and final category of the M3 Model is MaTTeR. Deep beneath the surface layers of our bodily experience are biochemical compounds that give the human body form and structure. These chemicals and molecules combine to produce the cells, tissues, organs, and structures that produce the symphony of life, behavior, performance, and disease that we experience. Now more than any other time in history, nearly anybody can get access to the deepest insights of their biochemical state. Genetic testing and blood work can provide precise data into the inner workings of the chemistry driving the mechanisms of performance longevity.

In this chapter, we'll explore how we got to this place of exquisite accuracy, some of the important indicators that might have an important place on your Performance Longevity Dashboard, and how to go about interpreting them. We'll also explore some proxy markers of biochemical health that may provide an accessible way to triangulate your overall biochemical state. As you read through this chapter, please remember that no indicator or tool discussed is meant to be a singular answer to any health or performance pursuit. Instead, they simply serve as a place to orient your attention so you can begin to actively explore an increased awareness of what's going on inside you and what tools may work to help you maintain or improve your path to health and performance.

Sending a vial of saliva to 23andMe or Ancestry.com to map your family tree or having blood drawn for health is commonplace in the twenty-first century, but even one hundred years ago, these things were a scientific revolution. Watson and Crick, the scientists responsible for discovering DNA, published their findings in the journal *Nature* on April 25, 1953— barely more than seventy years ago. In the span of just a few generations, we went from having an ambiguous idea of genetics, let alone their impact on disease, to pervasive public consciousness of the basic concept that genes play a major role in our ability to perform well and stay healthy.

Everybody knows the first step to becoming a professional athlete is to choose the right parents. It's not the only thing that counts, but, as big-wave surfing legend Laird Hamilton says, "There's chickens and there's hawks. You might not be able to turn a chicken into a hawk, but you can make a super chicken." Genetic testing has begun to give us an additional layer of preventative medicine as well. If we know what predispositions we have, it's possible to stay ahead of the game so we don't tempt fate with bad behavior.

It isn't as if humans weren't lifting the hood on the deeper causes of health and disease before the twentieth century. Many traditions around the globe have attempted to explain the unseen specters of performance and longevity for hundreds, if not thousands, of years. Traditional Chinese Medicine seeks to balance chi, the vital energy of the body, through diet, exercise, and interventions such as acupuncture and herbal medicine. Ayurvedic medicine from India works with doshas, categories that reveal energetic balance in mind and body also represented by various vital organs, bodily functions, and even attitudinal dispositions and emotions. Both Traditional Chinese Medicine and Ayurveda continue to be practiced by people all over India and China along with modern Western medicine. In ancient Greece, the state of the body was thought to be determined by the balance of the four elements as represented by the four humors: yellow (fire), black (earth) bile, phlegm (water), and blood (air). This theory of medicine was prevalent for two millennia, and even though anatomists like Andreas Vesalius challenged the core of these ideas, they influenced medical thinking into relatively recent history. Bloodletting, a common practice of physicians who ascribed to the Four Humors, was used

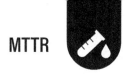

until the last decade of the nineteenth century, the same time the light bulb and telephone were invented.

The late 1800s and early 1900s gave rise to the discovery and understanding of enzymes, substances that speed up chemical reactions in the body, as well as leaps in regard to grasping metabolism. These might not sound exciting at first, but without an understanding of these components of our physiology, the effects of things like nutrition, medications, and exercise would be impossible to truly decipher. The 1940s and '50s were a golden age of biochemistry that propelled us toward the current era of precision medicine we have now. Although blood analysis was technically available in the 1800s, it was exceedingly expensive and unreliable. It wasn't until the 1950s that Leonard Skeggs invented the AutoAnalyzer and blood testing could be scaled.

Fast-forward to today, when relatively cheap and easy access to our biomarkers is more widely available than ever. We can get our blood drawn and analyzed without a doctor's note. That data can be input into apps on our smartphones that tell us how we should be eating to optimize our chemistry. We have monitors that can read our blood glucose levels in real time, watches that tell us our heart rates, and rings that know how well we sleep. We have DNA testing services that report our genetic heritage so we know what kinds of illnesses we might get. We have science that can tell us how bioavailable the nutrients in our food might be. We can measure our body composition in our own bathrooms.

On one hand, these technological tools are, in a word, miraculous. They allow for a level of precision in healthcare that was previously impossible. Health data, when used properly, can reveal hidden truths we otherwise would have learned about only at the point of failure. For example, early detection of genes that predispose women to breast cancer is possible, and there are blood markers that can help identify insulin resistance leading to type 2 diabetes far earlier than even a decade or two ago. Miraculous indeed.

On the other hand, it's easy to drown in the sea of data that's available. You get a blood test done. One doctor tells you to worry, while another says your markers are no big deal. One nutritionist says to eat meat, and another one says it will kill you. One exercise guru tells you to lift weights; another says you should go for walks instead. This abundance of information but lack of continuity can create confusion and frustration. Even worse, some charlatans in the field of health use this confusion to hornswoggle us into buying products we don't need or doing things that might even hurt us. You'd be surprised by how many people feel this lack of clarity. I have worked with professional athletes, C-suite executives, and elite soldiers, and they are often just as puzzled as everybody else in spite of their resources. Sometimes even more so because they have access to an even greater amount of information and even more people vying for their attention.

There are certainly biochemical indicators that are important for long-term performance and health and belong on the dashboard. At least as important, though, are the more proximal tools and indicators that deliver simple and reliable information that helps you make practical decisions to improve your life.

SELF-REFLECTION QUESTIONS

Take a moment to think about what you've learned so far about calibrating perception by using better indicators and tools. Now let's apply those same concepts to the category of MTTR.

Can you think of a situation where you ignored an indicator related to MTTR?

_____

_____

Were you unaware of the indicator, did you interpret it incorrectly, or did you just disregard it?

_____

_____

What happened as a result?

_____

_____

ALPHABET SOUP

Testosterone, estrogen, blood count, cholesterol, hemoglobin A1C, let's talk about your ApoB—"We didn't start the fi-re!" (Any Billy Joel fans out there?) The biomarkers available for measurement and analysis number in the thousands. The organic chemistry of living organisms, especially humans, can be complicated if not downright confounding. More and more books, podcasts, and services aim to harness the ease of twenty-first-century access to our biomarkers in an effort to optimize the chemistry that drives health and performance. For a layperson—heck, for anybody who hasn't deeply studied biochemistry—it can be difficult, if not impossible, to make sense of the alphabet soup of information when it comes to nutrition, supplements, and the types of exercise we are supposed to do to maintain our health. One of the downsides of the sea of available information is that it's easy to get exposed to conflicting opinions.

For this reason, I am not going to discuss all of the different chemical compounds and the stuff they do in this chapter. One thing I've noticed over the years is that while most people want to know that there is a scientific, biochemical rationale for the thing they're doing, most of us don't have a deep enough understanding of biochemistry to make heads or tails of it anyhow. We outsource that to people with more education on the subject. I certainly do. That's fine, because this book isn't about that. This book is about information suitable for a dashboard. Dashboards are about gleaning the most actionable information possible from data so that we can use to make decisions and then execute on them. That's what we're going to focus on here. That said, everything we will discuss comes from real consensus-driven research that can easily be found by referring to the resources section of this book or by performing a search on Google Scholar.

HIDDEN TRUTHS

Getting regular blood work can and should be an essential part of your Performance Longevity Dashboard. *Wait, Rob, didn't you just say that you're not gonna talk about this stuff?* Kind of. I'm not going to talk about specific blood markers in terms of values or ranges or what you should do about them. There are better resources for that kind of information than this book. What is important is that you look in the first place. Blood work shows you things that are hidden from the naked eye and provides a level of granularity and precision that you cannot achieve any other way. It shows you hidden truths about how your biology is responding to the cocktail of your genetics, behavior, and environment.

Basic, inexpensive yearly health panels are available from places like Thorne, Labcorp, InsideTracker, and Let's Get Checked and can go a long way toward keeping you from steering into blind spots. To dig into the deep details, you may need the help of a physician or other trusted healthcare practitioner. These direct-to-consumer panels are by no means perfect and certainly don't provide the same level of insight as some concierge medical practices. These are practices that offer private personalized, on-call services. They may also include other services, such as specially designed nutraceuticals—custom dietary supplements made to the specifications of your unique blood work—as well as a stable of in-house specialty health and performance experts.

Blood markers and even genetic testing as part of a comprehensive physical exam are pretty new but are becoming more and more commonplace. One of the persistent challenges that remains, and the primary benefit of access to things like concierge medicine, is having a trustworthy interpreter of this information. Remember, most physicians are trained under the

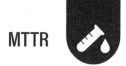

fundamental directive of illness correction, not performance longevity. Furthermore, most of the medical training offered in the last forty years has incentivized pharmaceutical intervention if a problem is detected. I'm not an anti-doctor or anti-pharmaceutical zealot by any stretch of the imagination. Both have saved my life on multiple occasions. But if you're uncertain about the interpretation of the data you're getting, seek help. Remember, you are the primary advocate for your own well-being, and you should never surrender it to anybody else. I know there are limits to my expertise and perspective, which means the same is true for everyone, regardless of the diploma on their wall. Once you find a person or resource you trust and who practices in a way that jibes with your goals and personality, stick with them as long as you get the results you want. Developing long-term relationships with your providers—people with relevant expertise who also work with you get to know your habits, rhythms, and dispositions—is important. This context is essential for making the best decisions possible to achieve performance longevity. The practitioners who help you interpret this essential information should know normative values (population-wide ranges), considerations for subpopulations (for example, if there are special considerations for people in your profession), and hopefully what is ideal for you as an individual. These layers taken together add valuable context to your biochemical data, especially over longer and longer timelines.

SELF-REFLECTION QUESTIONS

Do you currently monitor any indicators from this category of the M3 Model—such as biomarkers obtained from undergoing blood work or from a wearable device? If so, name a few examples.

What insight do those indicators provide?

Did you start to track them in response to a negative health event or as a precautionary measure?

_____

_____

Have you connected them to any specific behaviors?

_____

_____

Did they cause you to change any behaviors related to performance longevity?

_____

_____

Can you think of any MTTR indicators that you may have let go for too long?

_____

_____

What are some examples of leading indicators that inform you about MTTR-related trends in your health and performance?

_____

_____

If you notice a negative trend, what tools do you deploy to change it? Name a specific instance from your past, or, if you don't have one, make up a hypothetical example.

_____

_____

Of the proxy markers outlined in this chapter, which one do you think you could most easily create a personal health experiment for?

_____

_____

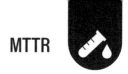

Name one marker for MTTR that you want to change. What metric will you use to measure your progress? Pick a tool that might affect this metric. State how often you would use it and for how long you would continue.

_____

_____

GOING DEEPER

The microscopic view of human health has had an enormously positive impact on the precision of both the leading indicators we use to prevent illness and the lagging indicators we use to measure the impact of the interventions we deploy. Hormones, genetics, and metabolic status can be measured inexpensively and at the click of a button (or more accurately, the tap of a screen). Far more meticulous measurements and therefore applications of medicine, nutrition, and sports science are available than ever before. It is performance optimization and medicine on a level of exactitude and scale that would have been hard to imagine even just ten or twenty years ago.

Computing and artificial intelligence aggregate and interpret health data at staggering speed and volume, allowing the health and performance industry to move forward at speeds that are hardly comprehensible. "Data is king" is on the banner of this data-driven revolution of industry, the benefits and trifles of which health information is an inseparable part. While the exponential pace of this technology allows for more accurate and granular measurements and descriptions of health and performance markers, some central problems remain.

First, even with the best access to measurement, how frequently is the average person collecting this data? Assuming you are getting blood work done once a year or even every six months for the explicit purpose of maintaining your health, there is still a significant gap in time for unwanted degradation in health and performance to occur. Many people still don't have regular access (or aren't using their access) to blood work at all. If they are, it's usually at the behest of a health practitioner once the engine is already smoking.

Once you collect this information, how can you make sense of it in a way that connects to actionable and sustainable changes in your behavior? In the tactical populations I work with, blood work information is often available but can be overwhelming in its complexity or, as I've observed, presented in a way that lacks cultural relevance. This can create a barrier to action for the end user—the very person it's meant to help.

In that case, which proxy markers for MTTR are valid, reliable, and easily accessible indicators of our biochemistry? Additionally, what fundamental, consistent health behaviors can collectively improve our biochemical profile?

Let's take a look.

HELPFUL PROXIES

Sophisticated forms of tracking indicators from the category of MTTR are certainly an important part of building your Performance Longevity Dashboard and Toolkit. However, what are more accessible proxy markers of biochemical health that are still valid and reliable? Furthermore, how can you use them to reasonably triangulate the state of your MTTR?

There are many topics I could choose to discuss in this section, but I've decided to focus on the three that seem the most prudent for performance longevity: sleep, aerobic health, and body composition. While these by no means cover every square inch of biochemistry, I focus on them in this chapter and again in the Personal Health Experiments that you will perform in the workbook for simple reasons.

First and foremost, they are based in rigorous science. None of these topics is even remotely controversial (famous last words in this day and age). Second, they are proximal! These indicators and tools are accessible

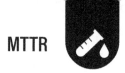

and relatively easy regardless of who you are and what kind of technology is available to you. To boot, any necessary interventions are easy to implement and learn from. Lastly, they yield large returns on investment. The indicators and tools we are going to look at are linchpin items in performance longevity and have stood the test of time as well.

A brief side note: Don't be fooled by the simplicity of these proxy markers. They are not intended to solve all health problems, nor are they necessarily intended to be medicinal. Instead, they are known bedrock factors in the long-term stability of health and performance. Even the highest-performing human beings on the planet need to be reminded of the importance of these simple but powerful indicators and interventions. A little-known secret of the high-performance world is that champions and warriors often perform in spite of poor health, not because of great health. Like the rest of us, they pay on the back end, and often in spades. Complexity bias can steer us to think that more complicated answers yield better solutions, but that is rarely true—not because life and health aren't complex but because complex problems with complicated solutions often make it much harder to be consistent with the things that solve the most problems.

Sleep: The Foundation of Biological Health

For most of human history, sleep was as natural as breathing. The rhythms of the sun dictated when people rose and when people rested, aligning their biological cycles with the rotation of the Earth. Circadian, from the Latin *circa dia* ("around a day"), describes these twenty-four-hour rhythms that regulate critical biochemical functions like metabolism, cognition, and, most importantly, sleep. Our internal clock is deeply embedded in our physiology, hardwired for a world where the setting sun signaled the approach of rest and the first light of dawn roused people into action.

Humans are, at our core, diurnal animals. Our physiology is built for wakefulness during daylight hours and recovery during the night. Think of it as a built-in gas pedal and brake system (see Chapter 4). Daylight presses the accelerator, fueling alertness and activity. Darkness gradually engages the brakes, slowing the system down in preparation for rest. For millennia, this cycle was automatic. The sun rose, and people woke. The sun set, and people slept.

But modernity has rewritten the script.

The world we've built no longer respects these ancient rhythms. We have outpaced our biology with a flood of artificial stimuli, the most obvious being light. It's not that people in the past never stayed up late—fires and candlelight allowed for nighttime activity. But today, we live in a perpetual daylight of our own making, one that disrupts the very system designed to regulate our sleep.

Meanwhile, the digital world keeps us engaged long past the point of fatigue, whether through doom-scrolling, late-night emails, or the endless availability of entertainment. We are no longer just ignoring our biological signals; we are actively overriding them.

The structure of modern life itself has shifted. The demands of late-night shifts, global work schedules, and an always-on culture have turned what was once an effortless biological process into something that now requires deliberate skill.

The consequence? Sleep, once automatic, is now something we must actively work to protect.

Sleep Deprivation Is Torture

The title of this section is not hyperbole. Prolonged sleep deprivation is so severe that it has been used as an interrogation technique. It's difficult to study the long-term effects of sleep deprivation because there are ethical limits on deliberately keeping people awake to observe when their systems begin to fail. (Even controlled sleep studies in labs are flawed—no one strapped to monitoring equipment in a sterile environment ever reports getting a great night's rest.)

What we do know is that sleep loss is stressful—not just mentally but also biologically. Even small reductions in sleep accumulate, affecting mood, decision-making, and physical health. Chronic sleep deprivation is linked to neurodegenerative diseases, cardiovascular issues, and metabolic dysfunction. Shift workers, who regularly disrupt their circadian rhythms, have a 26 percent higher likelihood of dying from coronary heart disease.

We don't need a scientific study to confirm that losing sleep makes us irritable, impulsive, and less effective. The modern world may demand more from us, but our biology doesn't care. The need for sleep remains nonnegotiable.

The Skill of Sleep: Relearning What Was Once Automatic

There are common rules of hygiene that we all accept: taking showers, brushing our teeth, and washing behind our ears—all of the stuff Mom made you do as a kid. Mom also said to go to bed on time, and she was right. Wouldn't it be weird if 40 percent of Americans reported that they didn't take enough showers? Or if people weren't brushing their teeth frequently enough, and at least once a month, their breath stank up their workplace? Sleep sometimes falls into a different category, though; while most of us do a decent job of keeping up with personal hygiene, we don't do so well with sleep hygiene, whether or not we realize it. That's probably because it's easier to tell when we haven't showered or brushed our teeth for a couple of days than it is to determine whether we are as well rested as we could be.

When I asked my clients over the years how they slept, most of them would answer, "Fine." Upon further investigation, sometimes with the help of wearable devices, we would discover that "fine" meant chronically unrested but used to it. Months or even years of suboptimal sleep reset our baseline expectations, making us think that feeling sluggish, foggy, and under-recovered is just part of life. But "fine" is not optimal. In fact, in March 2022 the U.S. Centers for Disease Control reported that 40 percent of Americans fall asleep during the day without meaning to at least once a month.

The good news? Sleep is a skill that can be learned.

To combat this ever-growing issue, sleep tracking functions are being installed in wearable rings, smartwatches, and even beds. All of this can be very helpful in bringing this important modulator of our physiology to the forefront of our minds and onto our dashboard. Before the cart, though, must come the horse. Answering a fundamental and often missed question can help elucidate the importance of sleep and what it is we are trying to accomplish.

What Is Sleep?

Everybody knows what sleep is, right? At least we think we do. "Rest," "repair," and "rebuilding" are words I often get when I ask attendees of Check Engine Light classes for their definitions of sleep. While these are correct in terms of outcomes, they don't get to the heart of what defines sleep. If we can define it accurately, it's much easier to measure it and then change it in ways that are simple, accessible, and impactful.

Sleep is not just being unconscious. Getting knocked out is clearly not the same thing as being asleep (no matter how loud the fight commentators yell, "He slept him!"). Natural sleep has definable behaviors that clearly differentiate it from other states of unconsciousness.

First, natural sleep usually occurs at night. Second, and more importantly, there are predictable and measurable cycles of behavior that occur in the brain and body during sleep. In general, these cycles, which I'll discuss in greater detail in the next section, occur every ninety to one hundred twenty minutes in adults between four and six times over the course of a night.

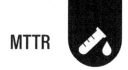

Understanding what sleep is and some of the normative values for sleep can help you make more informed decisions to maximize your much needed rest.

The Role of REM and NREM Sleep

During REM sleep, the brain exhibits high-frequency electrical waves similar to those of wakefulness, supporting cognitive and emotional functions.

- **Memory and emotional processing:** REM sleep plays a critical role in consolidating memories and regulating emotional reactivity. Research shows that REM sleep deprivation can impair emotional recognition and increase susceptibility to anxiety and mood disorders.

- **Neuromuscular calibration:** There is evidence that REM sleep helps refine motor control and spatial memory, particularly during early development. However, while REM sleep may play a role in motor learning, the exact mechanisms are still under investigation.

NREM sleep consists of both light and deep sleep stages, each with distinct functions.

- **Light sleep (stage 2 NREM):** Often overlooked, light sleep makes up about 50 percent of total sleep time. It includes the production of sleep spindles, bursts of neuronal activity thought to support memory consolidation and sensory processing. Scientists continue to explore the full significance of sleep spindles, but they appear to be critical for cognitive function.

- **Deep sleep (slow-wave sleep, or SWS):** The most restorative stage of sleep, deep sleep is vital for tissue repair, immune function, and cognitive health. During this stage:

  - The brain undergoes synaptic pruning, removing redundant neural connections to optimize learning and memory.

  - The body releases growth hormone, essential for muscle recovery and cellular repair.

- The lymphatic system flushes out metabolic waste, including proteins linked to neurodegenerative diseases.

There is some speculation that the default mode network (DMN)—the brain's background system for processing information and consolidating memories—may play a role in sleep-related cognition. While the DMN is highly active during wakeful rest, its precise function during sleep remains a topic of ongoing research.

Oft-Forgotten Latency

Sleep latency—the time it takes to transition from wakefulness to sleep—is a critical but often overlooked measure of sleep health. Ideally, falling asleep should take ten to twenty minutes, reflecting a well-regulated sleep drive and circadian alignment. Extremely fast sleep onset (under five minutes) may indicate chronic sleep deprivation, while prolonged sleep latency (over thirty minutes) can suggest poor sleep hygiene, stress, or circadian misalignment. Understanding sleep latency offers insight into overall sleep efficiency and nervous system regulation, making it a useful tool for assessing sleep quality.

Latency is closely tied to autonomic nervous system function, with elevated sympathetic (fight-or-flight) activity prolonging the time it takes to fall asleep. Techniques such as breathwork, meditation, and pre-bed relaxation can activate the parasympathetic (rest-and-digest) response, helping to shorten latency and promote deeper sleep. Sleep latency also influences sleep architecture—delayed onset can reduce total sleep time, increase nighttime awakenings, and shift REM sleep later into the night, disrupting its natural progression.

To maintain optimal sleep latency, consistency is key. A regular sleep schedule strengthens circadian rhythms, while limiting stimulants like caffeine and blue light exposure in the evening reduces sleep-onset delays. Creating a wind-down routine—incorporating reading, breathwork, or gentle movement—can further ease the transition into sleep. By monitoring and refining sleep latency, you can enhance overall sleep efficiency, improve recovery, and support long-term cognitive and physical health.

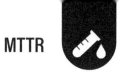

Sleep Synergy

If you take one thing away from this section, let it be this: Every stage of sleep matters. There's no single "most important" phase—the component pieces coalesce and synergize in an effort to reboot mind and body. This is especially important to remember when you track sleep information. It's okay to focus on improving a particular phase for a short time, but don't forget to zoom back out to the big picture.

Modern life, with all its artificial stimuli and disruptions, makes maintaining quality sleep more challenging. But by understanding the mechanics of sleep and developing strategies to protect it, you can regain control over this critical aspect of health.

Tracking sleep, adjusting your behaviors, and making informed choices can transform sleep from something you take for granted into something you actively optimize. Learning to navigate and fine-tune your sleep habits isn't just about feeling more rested—it's about sustaining performance, longevity, and overall well-being.

After all, our biology hasn't changed. But the world has. And if you want to keep up, you need to develop the skill of sleep.

First Responder/Tactical Work/Shift Work

If you work at odd hours, the ideals of sleep perfection can be annoying and anxiety-producing and may seem downright impossible. My work with first responders and military personnel has shown me how fatalistic people can become when they are constantly presented with an unattainable ideal. To you, I will quote the twenty-sixth president of the United States, Teddy Roosevelt: "Do what you can. When you can. With what you've got." It's not about making every night of sleep perfect. That's not realistic for anybody. Instead, strive to be as consistent as possible with the tools and opportunities that are available to you.

If you know that you are at a serious disadvantage either by the nature of your work or due to a temporary life event, then it behooves you to stack the deck as much in your favor as you possibly can, however you can. If you work the night shift, take hits to the head, or get exposed to toxic chemicals, is it more or less important to safeguard the primary biological activity your body uses to heal itself? Look back at the previous paragraphs, see what you *can* do, and start with that. My experience has shown me that the more you do what you can, the more you'll be able to do.

Gauging Restfulness: Indicators for Sleep

As I fine-tune this section, I'm struck by the potential obviousness of some of the information I've presented. The importance of sleep is more a part of public consciousness than ever. When I work with clients now, it's not that they don't realize they should be sleeping more and better; it's that they're not exactly sure how to measure their sleep and then alter the path they're on with some reasonable effect. Which brings us back to the whole point of this book: building a dashboard that makes sense for your vehicle and the way you want to drive it.

There are a few ways to go about tracking sleep. I'll cover those briefly here and then revisit them in the workbook.

Polysomnography (PSG)

Polysomnography, better known as a sleep study, is the gold standard for assessing sleep health. Typically conducted in a sleep laboratory or hospital, it provides a deep dive into the body's nighttime rhythms, using multiple

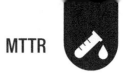

physiological measurements to evaluate sleep patterns and uncover potential disorders. It's usually reserved for individuals experiencing chronic sleep disturbances—those struggling with insomnia, sleep apnea, or other conditions that warrant closer investigation.

A sleep study unfolds under the watchful eye of trained specialists who monitor patients overnight, gathering data from a series of biometric sensors. Electroencephalography, or EEG, measures brainwave activity to track the stages of sleep, while electrooculography follows the movement of the eyes, particularly during REM sleep. Muscle activity is recorded through electromyography, capturing subtle shifts in tone and movement throughout the night. The heart's rhythm and rate are assessed via electrocardiography, and respiratory sensors combined with pulse oximetry provide crucial insight into airway function, breathing patterns, and blood oxygen levels. Together, these tools create a comprehensive picture of how a person sleeps, offering valuable clues that can lead to formal diagnoses and targeted treatment plans.

Despite its reputation as the most accurate method for analyzing sleep, polysomnography comes with its own set of challenges. Many patients report difficulty sleeping in a lab setting, particularly during the first night. This common phenomenon, known as the first-night effect, reflects a temporary decline in sleep quality due to the unfamiliar environment and the sensation of being hooked up to monitoring equipment. It's something I've heard echoed time and again from clients who've undergone sleep studies— many say they slept even worse than usual, despite being accustomed to poor sleep at home.

In recent years, advancements in wearable technology and portable monitoring devices have made at-home sleep studies a viable alternative for some people. While these at-home setups lack the controlled conditions of a laboratory, they offer a level of comfort that might actually improve compliance and provide a more realistic snapshot of a person's typical sleep patterns. Still, for those in need of the most precise data, the traditional in-lab study remains the best option, offering an unparalleled window into the complexities of sleep.

Hypnograms

Hypnograms are charts that plot out the phases of sleep over the course of the night. Lots of wearable devices offer hypnograms along with summaries of the information presented. This data is compared against known normative values for sleep behavior. For example, in the image that follows, you can see the normative representation of falling asleep, and then the first and longest cycle of deep sleep, as well as the stages of light sleep that buttress the transition to increasing time in REM. While very few, if any, of us fit perfectly into this schematic, these norms offer a North Star to begin navigating by. More importantly, hypnograms can provide measurable insight into how different behaviors either improve or detract from the sleep your body needs to reset and rejuvenate itself. These more precise sleep indicators can help you calibrate your perception and make more informed choices about your sleep habits over time.

Beware, though; these devices are not perfect, and the summaries may require deeper investigation. As a recent personal example, I woke up one morning after what I thought was a restful night of sleep. Upon inspection of my Ōura app, I saw that I had a mere twenty-eight minutes of deep sleep compared to my normal hour and twenty to thirty minutes! *What happened?!* I wondered. I went to bed on time. I didn't stare at a brightly lit screen or drink alcohol before bed. I wasn't noticeably stressed. Further investigation revealed a gap in the data during my second sleep cycle. *No sleep* was recorded for a period of time in the middle of the night. My ring must have spun around on my finger, rendering an incomplete data set that showed up on the graph but not in my sleep summary. Most of my second cycle of deep sleep was not accounted for. It turns out I had slept just fine. In other words, don't simply take the data you receive at face value; dig a little deeper to make sure things are as they seem.

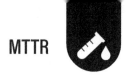
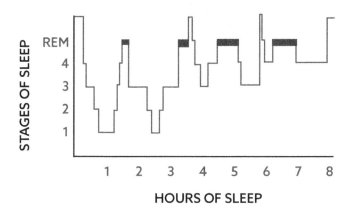

HOURS OF SLEEP

Internal Reviews

The most accessible indicator of sleep loss is—wait for it—feeling tired. While I say this partially tongue-in-cheek, internal reviews can be great tools for enhancing your awareness of your rest. Sleep questionnaires like the ones you'll use in some experiments in the workbook can inspire you to ask yourself important questions about how rested you feel and help you connect with your behavior in many of the same ways that hypnograms can.

Sleep questionnaires, like the Sleep Quality Scale shown here, are statistically reliable surveys used to assess sleep. You can download this one online and use it to test your own sleep hypotheses, or pick a few of the points that are most relevant to you and ask yourself those questions when you wake up in the morning.

Sleep Quality Scale Examples	
Rarely	None or 1–3 times a month
Sometimes	1–2 times a week
Often	3–5 times a week
Almost always	6–7 times a week

Sleep Quality Scale	Rarely	Sometimes	Often	Almost always
I have difficulty falling asleep.	O	O	O	O
I fall into a deep sleep.	O	O	O	O
I wake up while sleeping.	O	O	O	O
I have difficulty getting back to sleep once I wake up in middle of the night.	O	O	O	O
I wake up easily because of noise.	O	O	O	O
I toss and turn.	O	O	O	O
I never go back to sleep after awakening during sleep.	O	O	O	O
I feel refreshed after sleep.	O	O	O	O
I feel unlikely to sleep after sleep.	O	O	O	O
Poor sleep gives me headaches.	O	O	O	O
Poor sleep makes me irritated.	O	O	O	O
I would like to sleep more after waking up.	O	O	O	O
My sleep hours are enough.	O	O	O	O
Poor sleep makes me lose my appetite.	O	O	O	O
Poor sleep makes it hard for me to think.	O	O	O	O
I feel vigorous after sleep.	O	O	O	O
Poor sleep makes me lose interest in work or others.	O	O	O	O
My fatigue is relieved after sleep.	O	O	O	O
Poor sleep causes me to make mistakes at work.	O	O	O	O
I am satisfied with my sleep.	O	O	O	O
Poor sleep makes me forget things more easily.	O	O	O	O
Poor sleep makes it hard to concentrate at work.	O	O	O	O
Sleepiness interferes with my daily life.	O	O	O	O
Poor sleep makes me lose desire in all things.	O	O	O	O
I have difficulty getting out of bed.	O	O	O	O
Poor sleep makes me easily tired at work.	O	O	O	O
I have a clear head after sleep.	O	O	O	O
Poor sleep makes my life painful.	O	O	O	O

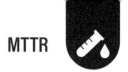
Like any metric, these kinds of reviews come with caveats. For example, as I mentioned at the beginning of this book, your own perception is not always reliable. As such, the thermostat for your state of normalcy can get skewed. When I work with people in the military special operations community and ask how they're feeling, they could be dragging their legs behind them with black circles under their eyes, but their answer is almost inevitably, "Good to go." While I most assuredly admire their tenacity, that kind of skewed feedback does not provide usable information for making long-term health and performance decisions.

So, what the heck, Rob? Wearables are good, but don't totally rely on them? Internal perception should be used, but don't rely on that, either? Now you're getting it. Don't put all your eggs in any one basket. Play these metrics against each other. Neither your perception nor your devices have all of the answers. But, as you bounce them back and forth, you will develop more clarity about the reality you're dealing with. As you develop your skill with this practice, you can go from clunky, slow reactions where you seem behind the eight ball, hoping you're getting good information and doing the right thing, to something much better: *tuning.* Just like tuning an instrument. Small adjustments that keep things playing nicely. More details on that in forthcoming chapters. Stay tuned. (Get it?)

Individual Factors

While there are definitely gutters in the bowling lane of sleep, the set of arrows you use to roll a strike might be different from the set another person uses. Chronotypes, genetics, hormonal fluctuations, and life rhythms all have a say in how much and how well you sleep.

Chronotypes are genetically predetermined times for sleep. While everybody needs the proverbial eight hours, *when* those eight hours should occur can vary from person to person. Morning types tend to fall asleep early and feel the most naturally alert earlier in the day, while night owls tend to fall asleep much later and wake later in morning, hitting their performance stride in the afternoon hours.

Age is another major player. Deep sleep declines as we get older, and circadian rhythms shift, making early wake-ups more common in older adults. Then there's genetics. Some people naturally need less sleep, while others are predisposed to conditions like insomnia or narcolepsy.

Hormones throw another wild card into the mix, especially for women. Menstrual cycles, pregnancy, and menopause can all disrupt sleep by influencing body temperature, melatonin production, and stress hormone levels. Fluctuations in estrogen and progesterone mean that some nights are restful while others feel like a wrestling match with the sheets.

Other individual factors, like preferred room temperatures and eating times, along with basic life stuff like your kids' school events or your own social needs, can play a role in the push and pull of how you organize appropriate rest for yourself. The point is that everybody is a little different. If you have good indicators to help you know where you stand, you can deploy the tools that work best for you and be adaptable as your needs change over time.

Sleep Tune-Up: Practical Tools for Better Sleep

Over-the-counter sleep aids are a booming industry, with the global market valued between $20 and $60 billion in 2022. Despite increasing awareness of the importance of sleep, many people still struggle to align their rest with modern life. Some argue that doing so is a matter of discipline, but the real issue lies in how we structure our behaviors. Our current systems aren't strong enough to counteract the subtle but pervasive habits that erode sleep quality. In other words, we don't always know which dials to turn or which tools will make a meaningful impact.

With countless sleep interventions and products vying for attention, it's easy to get lost in the noise. While some solutions can be helpful, the key to consistently better sleep isn't found in a pill bottle or an expensive gadget—it's in understanding and leveraging fundamental biological principles. The most effective way to improve sleep isn't through quick fixes but by developing a skill set that allows you to adjust your environment and behavior in ways that promote reliable, restful sleep.

First, you'll learn about the strategies I refer to as stable levers—the nonnegotiable factors that influence sleep, rooted in human biology and circadian rhythms. Unlike fleeting sleep hacks, stable levers remain consistent across different circumstances. Learning to identify and manipulate these factors gives you more control over your sleep, no matter your situation. Then we'll look at other factors that can influence sleep health, such as exercise, enrichment activities, and even alternative ways to improve rest when sleep isn't available.

Note that you don't need to overhaul everything at once. Some changes may not be feasible in your current routine, and that's okay. The goal is to make gradual, measurable adjustments—one at a time—while tracking their effects. Over time, these small tweaks compound, helping you fine-tune your sleep in a way that works for you.

Stable Levers

Light

Light is the strongest circadian lever you can pull. Your brain uses light exposure to determine when you should be alert and when you should wind down. The retina connects directly to the suprachiasmatic nucleus (SCN) in the hypothalamus, which acts as your body's master clock. Morning and evening light exposure help anchor this clock, reinforcing a stable sleep cycle.

What helps:

- Consistent natural light exposure (ten to thirty minutes outside in the morning and five to ten minutes at sunset) strengthens circadian rhythms and optimizes melatonin production.

- Reducing blue light exposure at night by dimming screens, using night mode, or shifting to warmer (red/orange) lighting signals to the body that night is approaching.

- Creating a dark sleep environment with blackout curtains or an eye mask enhances sleep quality.

- Wearing blue-light-blocking glasses (with amber-colored lenses) can be moderately effective if screen use at night is unavoidable—just ensure they actually block blue light (if you can still see the color blue, they aren't working).

What hurts:

- Blue light exposure (from screens and artificial lighting) within two to three hours of bedtime disrupts melatonin production.

- Bright LED lights at night, even if warm-toned, can suppress melatonin if too intense.

- Inconsistent light exposure throughout the day weakens circadian alignment, making it harder to fall asleep and wake up refreshed.

There certainly is a menu of items for pulling the lever of light to affect your sleep. The most important thing, regardless of the one you choose at any time, is to remain aware that the light you are being exposed to is powerfully affecting your body's clock. Know what signal you're getting and then change it if need be to achieve the outcomes you want.

Temperature

The next sleep lever is temperature. Cooling the environment and the cooling of your core body temperature are essential aspects of falling and staying asleep. Too hot or too cold has been shown to cause restlessness during sleep that interrupts dense, natural cycles of rest. Lower core body temperatures synchronize you with your first light sleep cycle and prepare your body to enter into deeper stages of restorative sleep. Let's take a look at what hurts and what helps when it comes to temperature.

What helps:

- **Cool room temperature (65°F to 70°F):** Adjust based on age, muscle mass, and preference.

- **Warm shower or bath 90 to 120 minutes before bed:** This triggers vasodilation, cooling core temperature as blood flows to the skin.

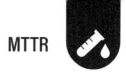

- **Breathable bedding and pajamas:** Prevent overheating, which disrupts deep sleep.

What hurts:

- **Late-night exercise:** Exercise elevates core body temperature, delaying sleep. While physical activity has been shown to improve sleep, research tends to indicate finishing exercise two to four hours prior to bedtime. If training late, stick to lower-intensity movement (e.g., walking or stretching).

- **Eating too close to bedtime:** Large, high-calorie meals increase body temperature, potentially delaying sleep onset and fragmenting sleep. For most, the effect is minimal, but it may contribute to further disruption in sleep-sensitive individuals.

- **Cold plunging before bed:** This can increase wakefulness due to a norepinephrine spike. If this is a part of your practice, do it earlier in the evening to allow for a cooling rebound.

Regardless of exactly how you decide to manipulate your sleep temperature, it's certainly a powerful and stable lever you can pull to move closer to the restorative sleep you need to feel and perform your best. My recommendation, as always, is to identify an outcome, try the tool, and measure the effect.

Nutrition

The timing of meals plays a crucial role in sleep quality, with eating too close to bedtime often leading to fragmented sleep. While the effects on total sleep duration and architecture are mixed, research suggests that late-night eating can disrupt the continuity of sleep, making it less restful overall. Additionally, it can have metabolic consequences that may further impact long-term sleep health.

What helps:

- Finishing meals at least three hours before bedtime allows digestion to settle and reduces sleep disturbances.

- Choosing lighter evening meals can prevent metabolic disruptions and minimize sleep fragmentation.

- Maintaining consistent meal timing supports circadian rhythm alignment, promoting better overall sleep quality.

- Avoiding high-sugar and high-fat foods late at night can help stabilize blood sugar levels, reducing the risk of sleep interruptions.

What hurts:

- Eating within one to three hours before bed increases sleep fragmentation, leading to more frequent nighttime waking.

- Late-night meals can cause a compensatory increase in sleep duration, but this does not necessarily improve sleep quality.

- Disrupted sleep patterns may lead to deeper sleep early in the night followed by lighter sleep later, reducing overall restfulness.

- Metabolic effects, such as elevated glucose levels and altered fat metabolism, can indirectly affect sleep quality over time.

By being mindful of when and what you eat in the evening, you can optimize both sleep duration and quality, ensuring more restorative rest.

The Ups and Downs of Caffeine, Nicotine, and Alcohol

Alcohol in any amount impairs restful sleep. There, I said it. Does this mean you can't drink and "sleep like a rock"? Nope. You can certainly tie one on and pass out pretty darn hard. But we already know that doesn't guarantee quality rest. Alcohol is especially detrimental to REM sleep. While the ol' hot toddy has been a sleep ritual for a very long time, it leads to sedation and not sleep in the strictest terms. Does it mean that if you have a drink before bed every night, your brain will turn to dust? No. But there is a price to be paid. Know that drinking

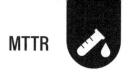

alcohol costs you and make a conscious choice about if and when you're willing to pay that price.

Caffeine and nicotine are two commonly ingested drugs that are known for their performance-enhancing qualities as well as their addictiveness. While they work on different pathways, the stimulating nature of these drugs can interfere with sleep onset and architecture. Not only that, but caffeine and nicotine are very often used as part of a dysfunctional cycle of stimulation and sedation that shields the user from the reality of their situation, particularly in fields that are high stress and require shift work.

When used responsibly, these compounds can be fun and even helpful in some cases, but when used in excess or with poor timing, they can be additional inhibitors to achieving the restoration your body and mind require.

Routine

Even if you have a routine in place, it may be counterproductive to your native physiology and create friction in the message you are trying to send. If your nightly pre-sleep protocol involves drinking a beer while you yell at the news, you are not helping your body prepare for rest. The same is true for looking at bright screens or answering emails.

Sleep hygiene around bedtime doesn't need to be complicated. When my daughter was little, every night about an hour before bed, she took a warm shower and then put on her jammies and read a bedtime story. It can be that simple for you, too, albeit with a bit more sophistication based on the things you're learning in this chapter. You'll have the chance to try some things that work for you in the Personal Health Experiments, too.

What helps:

- **Consistent sleep-wake timing:** Strengthens circadian alignment. Inconsistent schedules create jet-lag effects, even without travel. On a personal note, I've found this simple behavioral change to have the highest-magnitude effect on both my sleep quality and my HRV.

- **Relaxation before bed:** Low-stimulation activities (such as reading, breathwork, and stretching) activate the parasympathetic nervous system, easing the transition to sleep.

- **Dimming lights and reducing screen time:** Minimizes melatonin suppression. Melatonin was the cat's pajamas in sleep aids for a hot minute, but if you're still exposing yourself to bright white light, you may be peeing upwind.

What hurts:

- **Alcohol before bed:** Shortens sleep onset but wrecks sleep architecture by fragmenting REM.

- **Doomscrolling or news consumption:** Overstimulates the brain, keeping cortisol high when it should be dropping.

Noise

Your evolutionary brain still reacts to unexpected sounds as potential threats. Sudden or inconsistent noises can fragment sleep, while consistent sound can improve it. With that said, there are some sounds that are clearly disruptive to our sleep. Obviously, the shrill tones of sirens and alarms will wake anybody from a sound slumber. That's sort of the point.

Moving toward as consistent an overall sleeping environment as possible is the name of the game.

What helps:

- **Pink noise:** Frequencies lower than white noise may enhance deep sleep. While pink noise shows some promise, including improving sleep security for surgical patients, there is lots of room for individual

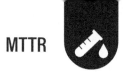

variability. Be sure to test for yourself, but focus on moving the big rocks first!

- **Binaural beats:** Binaural beats, created by presenting slightly different frequencies to each ear, may enhance sleep quality, though effects vary by frequency and individual response.

- **Nature sounds (rain, ocean waves):** These can be more relaxing than white noise. While the exact mechanisms are unclear, some nature sounds can induce relaxation and improve sleep latency.

- **Earplugs or soundproofing:** If you live near heavy traffic or loud neighbors, this is a game changer.

What hurts:

- **Road traffic, railway, and air traffic noise:** These types of sounds seem to be the most disruptive to sleep.

- **Loud or unfamiliar noises:** If you're in an unfamiliar environment with distracting noises (like the banging of hotel room doors combined with a powerful HVAC system kicking on), it may be helpful to block them out if possible.

- **Stimulating music or sounds:** While there isn't direct evidence that music has a substantial negative impact on sleep, increasing arousal certainly won't help.

These stable levers by no means offer the entire kit and caboodle, but they are accessible starting points to manipulate your sleep. Be sure to check out the Personal Health Experiments section at the back of this book so you can start investigating what works best for you.

Supplements

Over-the-counter sleep supplements are in use more now than ever before. One could write a whole book on this subject alone, but let's touch on some of the supplements that are safe to run personal experiments with, won't hurt your ability to truly rest or cause dependency, and of course, have displayed actual efficacy. Any supplement is just that—a supplement. My suggestion is to rely on the stable levers (robust and proximal tools) as your first line of offense in improving your sleep.

One of the interesting things about sleep supplements is that regardless of the mechanism, they all have a similar outcome: pumping the brakes on your nervous system (Chapter 4 callback!). Common sleep agents like magnesium, valerian root, and L-theanine all work to regulate gamma-aminobutyric acid (GABA). GABA is the brain's primary inhibitory neurotransmitter responsible for slowing down nervous system activation and promoting relaxation. Essentially, all sleep supplements encourage your nervous system to chill out—something to keep in mind when you think about other, more proximal tools that could be included in your sleep toolkit.

Exercise Is Key

Exercise does not solve all of life's problems, but it sure seems to help with most of them, including sleep. Regular physical activity is consistently linked to improved sleep quality, but the type, intensity, and timing of exercise all play a role in how much it helps (or hinders) rest.

Aerobic exercise, particularly moderate-intensity activity like jogging, cycling, and swimming, appears to be the most effective at promoting deeper sleep and aiding recovery from sleep loss. Resistance training has also been shown to enhance sleep efficiency over time, though its effects on sleep onset can vary. High-intensity workouts, especially late in the evening, can be a double-edged sword—while some individuals report improved sleep, others experience elevated heart rate, core body temperature, and sympathetic nervous system activation, all of which can delay sleep onset.

Timing matters. Exercising at least three to four hours before bed gives your body time to cool down and shift into a parasympathetic state, making sleep more accessible. That said, individual responses vary—some people fall asleep easily after late-night workouts, while others find them disruptive. The key is experimentation: Identify an outcome, track how different workouts affect your sleep, and adjust accordingly. If you're not sure where to start, get guidance—and stay tuned for the sleep experiments in the workbook.

There is growing evidence that regular exercise is conducive to a good night's rest. Moderate exercise a few hours before bed may be especially beneficial for people who have trouble getting to sleep at night. While aerobic exercise seems to be the most conducive to both getting to sleep and recovering from sleep loss, researchers have not yet reached a clear consensus on what type, how much, and for whom different flavors of exercise will help with sleep. How do you know which kind might help you and which kind might not? Do an experiment! Identify an outcome, assign a measurement, find a type and amount of exercise you know won't hurt you, and try it. If you're not sure where to start, get help—and stay tuned for the experiments in the workbook.

Rest Is Second Best

There are times in life when getting great sleep just isn't in the cards. You work at night, you have a new baby, you're a stressed entrepreneur, or maybe your dog had surgery and keeps knocking his stupid cone against the wall and waking you up. Whatever the reason, it can help to have a few aces up your sleeve to recoup some rest. As a caveat, none of these is a replacement for a full night of sleep.

- **Pump the brakes:** Yep, this again. While inducing a parasympathetic state is not the same as going through the restorative cycles of sleep, it can help reboot your nervous system when you need it. Breathing exercises, meditation, and progressive relaxation exercises are reliable ways to pump the brakes for a few minutes and let your brain and body recharge.

- **Self-induced hypnagogic states:** Hypnagogia is a transitional state of consciousness that naturally occurs between wakefulness and sleep. Creatives like Salvador Dali and Thomas Edison were known for harnessing this condition (hypoid state) by falling asleep with objects in their hands that would fall out and make noise, waking them during this heightened state of relaxation and creativity.

- **Autogenic training (AT) and Yoga Nidra:** These are effective non-pharmacological techniques for improving sleep and relaxation. AT uses self-induced relaxation to reduce stress and enhance sleep quality, particularly in those with insomnia. Yoga Nidra, a guided meditation, promotes deep rest by increasing total sleep time and efficiency while reducing insomnia symptoms. Both methods support relaxation through physiological and psychological mechanisms. AT calms the nervous system, while Yoga Nidra increases delta brainwave activity, mimicking deep sleep. By reducing stress and improving sleep architecture, these practices offer accessible tools for better rest and overall well-being.

- **Naps:** Naps can enhance mood, reduce fatigue, and improve cognitive performance, with benefits observed across various age groups. The effectiveness of a nap depends on its duration and timing, with short (around thirty-minute) naps in the early afternoon offering the greatest benefits while minimizing sleep inertia. Individual differences, such as age and habitual napping behavior, influence how restorative a nap can be, making personal experimentation key to optimizing results.

If you find yourself in a pinch, you can pull any of these tools out of your bag to keep yourself on the road. Be sure to test them before you need them to find which are the most robust, reliable, and repeatable for you.

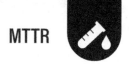

Seek Enrichment

In addition to behaviors near sleep that help set you up for improved rest are the cycles of behavior that you engage in all day long. Your circadian sleep clock doesn't start an hour before bedtime; it starts when you wake up from the previous night of sleep. The things you do all day long, your total stress load, and the ways you do or don't use your body can have important effects on your ability to rest. If you've met your basic needs through some enriching interaction with your environment, it can be easier to enter into states of rest with less agitation. The study of this subject is still new and, at the time I did research for this book, is limited to mice, but anecdotally it rings true in my experience. Take that for what it's worth.

Environmental enrichment is used for animals in captivity to make their living space more dynamic, complex, and stimulating and has been found to reverse maternal sleep deprivation in mice. Captive animals who do not engage in enrichment-based activities have a far greater likelihood of behavioral dysfunction and health problems. Everybody knows that if you take your dog for a walk at a new park, the dog sleeps like the dead afterward. Why? The dog's brain has to process all of that novel environmental information. It stands to reason that some of that evolutionary residue is stuck to us as well. I know nothing makes me sleep better than spending a day outside in the sun doing chores at the horse barn. No sleep supplement, foam rolling, or breathwork has ever had the same positive effect as getting outside and moving my body around. It's like that's what we're made to do or something…

 THE POWER OF ENRICHMENT

Client R is a professional coach. I won't say which sport in an effort to keep their identity private. When I started to work with R, one of their main goals was to improve both the quality and the quantity of their sleep. For at least a decade, this person had struggled to get to sleep and stay asleep, and even when they did, they often did not feel well rested when they woke. Every week or so, however, they would hit a level of exhaustion that would collapse them into a ten- or eleven-hour night of slumber that would reboot the system just enough to keep getting by. Needless to say, this cycle was having a deleterious effect on their mental and physical gas tanks.

When we discussed what sleep interventions they had tried, the list was a long one of trial, error, and frustration to the point of fatalistic acceptance. Sleep supplements like magnesium, L-theanine, and melatonin (a hot commodity at one point that is now mostly recommended against), as well as pharmaceuticals prescribed by physicians. Meditations, eye masks, essential oil diffusers. The list went on and on. Nothing seemed to be working.

On a hunch, I asked R to take the Big Five Personality Test. I knew that R was highly intelligent, but it turned out that they were also very high in trait Openness, a predictor of aesthetic sensitivity and creative drive. For people high in this trait, creation is a need, not a fun thing to do on rare occasion. As it turned out, R had not been engaged in any creative behavior outside of coaching for years. They had a fundamental need that was not being met. Their enrichment did not match their needs.

I recommended two things: First, a creative endeavor, in this case Morning Pages (refer to Chapter 4). Second, a daily walk with no expressed goal—just wander around and think. While these two interventions were not enough to fully resolve R's sleep issues, they did make a difference. R now experiences far fewer difficulties with sleep, often achieving a consistent seven to eight hours a night. More importantly, they have developed a deeper understanding of their own enrichment needs and the connection between seemingly unrelated behaviors and sleep quality. Everything is interconnected—there is only one big picture.

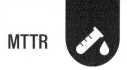

Sleep Tight

Sleep is an essential biological activity and an important indicator for performance longevity. This discussion has been a very brief overview of the importance of this marker and the implications it has for staying your best for as long as you can. Knowing that it's important to get good-quality sleep is one thing, but getting it is another thing altogether. If you struggle with this aspect of your health, I urge you to make it a priority. I cannot overstate the positive effect that it will have on both your immediate performance and your long-term health.

The negative effects of chronic sleep loss may be subtle and pervasive. The nefarious little weeds that sprout from this issue may not be obvious at first, but like rust collecting on your muffler, one day the whole thing just falls off. Sleep, like all human biology, is complex, but getting it right doesn't need to be complicated. Keep things simple by relying on stable levers. It is not essential to get every single thing right all the time. Instead, think in terms of net outcomes and "do what you can, when you can, with what you've got" to make slow, steady improvements.

Body Composition: Body Fat and Muscle Mass

We are at a point in human evolution where we have become so biologically successful that not only is there a surplus of food in most of the world, but many of us carry some of that surplus on our bodies. It is more and more common for people to be overweight and even obese. Sometimes ideas of body positivity get conflated with ideas of health. Being overweight or obese does not reduce your value as a person. Some of the best people I've ever known were overweight or obese. They were intelligent, kind, compassionate, wonderful people. But they were not healthy. Some of them tragically died earlier and more brutally from causes that are largely preventable with lifestyle changes.

Guess what? I've had plenty of unhealthy habits, too. I just didn't have to wear them for the whole world to see and talk about. So let's change this conversation from one based on value judgment to one that's about formulating plans to solve problems. While much of the time the discussion of obesity conflates weight with aesthetics rather than health, an easily demonstrable fact remains: There are stable ranges of body fat and, at least equally important, muscle mass that support performance longevity. Body composition, which is the ratio of fat to lean tissue, is an accessible marker that provides clear insight into health.

Let's get clear on something right away: Being overweight doesn't mean you can't perform well. In some sports, like powerlifting and sumo wrestling, packing on pounds can be an asset and is sometimes even encouraged. What most people don't know is that behind the scenes in those sports, there are a lot of CPAP machines. Being overweight doesn't necessarily mean you won't live a long time, either. We all have that one uncle who lived until he was seventy-nine even though he was overweight, smoked half a pack of cigarettes, and drank a six-pack a day. But it means the burden on your body to perform well and sustain life will be predictably more significant. When it comes to health, there are no free lunches. You pay up front or you pay on the back end. But either way you pay, and paying on the back end often comes with accrued interest.

Ideal body composition falls within reasonable ranges that vary primarily by age and sex. Men have an essential body fat percentage of about 3 percent, while for women, it's around 12 percent. Falling below these essential levels can lead to metabolic and endocrine dysfunction. Athletes as a group tend to be leaner than non-athletes, but striving for an athletic body composition can benefit everyone. Maintaining lower levels of body fat—particularly visceral fat (fat stored around the organs)—while preserving or even increasing muscle mass is a strong predictor of performance longevity. Excess visceral fat, in particular, is linked to a higher risk of all-cause mortality, including cardiovascular disease and metabolic syndrome.

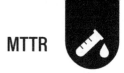

Fitness Categories for Body Composition (% Body Fat) for Men by Age							
%		Age (in years)					
		20-29	30-39	40-49	50-59	60-69	70-79
99	Very lean	4.2	7.3	9.5	11.1	12.0	13.6
95		6.4	10.3	13.0	14.9	16.1	15.5
90		7.9	12.5	15.0	17.0	18.1	17.5
85	Excellent	9.1	13.8	16.4	18.3	19.2	19.0
80		10.5	14.9	17.5	19.4	20.2	20.2
75		11.5	15.9	18.5	20.2	21.0	21.1
70	Good	12.6	16.8	19.3	21.0	21.7	21.6
65		13.8	17.7	20.1	21.7	22.4	22.3
60		14.8	18.4	20.8	22.3	23.0	22.9
55		15.8	19.2	21.4	23.0	23.6	23.6
50	Fair	16.7	20.0	22.1	23.6	24.2	24.1
45		17.5	20.7	22.8	24.2	24.9	24.5
40		18.6	21.6	23.5	24.9	25.6	25.2
35		19.8	22.4	24.2	25.6	26.4	25.7
30	Poor	20.7	23.2	24.9	26.3	27.0	26.3
25		22.1	24.1	25.7	27.1	27.9	27.1
20		23.3	25.1	26.6	28.1	28.8	28.0
15		25.1	26.4	27.7	29.2	29.8	29.3
10	Very poor	26.6	27.8	29.1	30.6	31.2	30.6
5		29.3	30.2	31.2	32.7	33.5	32.9
1		33.7	34.4	35.2	36.4	37.2	37.3
n=		1,938	10,457	16,032	9,976	3,097	571

Maintaining body composition is accomplished through a reasonable attendance to diet and regular and organized movement of the body. In practice, it's not much more complicated than that, but people who sell products have a vested interest in making it seem like it is. Not to beat the drum of complexity bias yet again, but we tend to think complex problems require complex answers, and the fact is that more often than not, they don't.

Caloric Budgeting

Modern life does throw some wrenches into the gears of this biological simplicity, though. For one, more calorically dense food is available to us than ever before. A pint of Ben & Jerry's ice cream, which I personally can take right to the face with ease, has around 1,200 calories. One time I went shopping with a family member who was trying to lose weight, and we looked at some of their favorite "bad day," "boredom," and "fun" foods. For this person, who is about 5'4", Ben & Jerry's was at the top of their list. We figured out that one pint of ice cream added more than a third to their reasonable range of required daily calories. And that was just one of the foods we identified.

Most of us do not have an accurate sense of food value. How could we? Our biological mechanisms for taste and satiety are not built to understand much of the food that is on grocery store shelves. That means unless we count calories or manage caloric load in some other way, we have no idea what's going in there. Many calorie-dense processed foods don't trigger satiety in the same way that whole foods often do. The fibrous content that helps trigger signals of satiety is removed, and we just get to stuffing. A pound of feathers and a pound of gold both weigh a pound, but there is a significant difference in their value. Moving toward real, whole foods as a rule is a good thing, but sometimes we have to read between the lines.

This inaccurate sense of food value can follow us right into healthy diets. I remember back in the early 2000s, when the Paleo diet was all the rage in CrossFit gyms, our CrossFit gym decided to do a Paleo diet challenge. One particular individual at the gym managed to gain over five pounds of fat during our 30-Day Paleo Challenge. When we asked him what he'd been eating, his Paleo food of choice turned out to be dehydrated fruit. This guy was literally eating entire bags of dried fruit every day. A dehydrated apple actually has more caloric content than a whole apple, but none of the water or fiber, so the signal of fullness doesn't arrive nearly as soon. One bag of dehydrated apples or mangoes might have eight to ten pieces of fruit in it. Try to sit down and eat eight apples in a row, I double-dog-dare you. Actually, I don't—the gastric distress might cost you a day of work. So essentially, this client of ours was eating bags of apples, mangoes, and bananas every week, adding up to thousands of excess calories. He earned the affectionate nickname Fruit Monkey, and it has stuck for years.

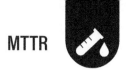

Wait, isn't Paleo healthy? It can be. As can many of the myriad diets and, perhaps a better term, nutritional styles. Once you control for calories, much of the nutritional style we choose boils down to personal preference. As is often the case, understanding what in the heck is really going on requires you to look more closely.

Nutrition is one of the most confusing and dare I say fervor-filled areas of health you can dive into. I know everybody thinks that their favorite flavor of ice cream is the best one and everybody else's is stupid, but it is just a fact that the things we argue over often come down to taste. What culture and communication style tickle the right feelings? When it comes to nutrition, I find it best to be agnostic. I couldn't care less what type of nutritional approach resonates with you. (The same goes for your flavor of exercise. Not everybody likes to throw heavy weights around.) If you like to eat Ayurvedic, that's fine. And if you do eat according to your doshas but you're still overweight or obese, guess what? The risk factors are the same regardless of which diet god you happen to pray to. The point is to legitimately attend to the essential factors that provide metrics you can manipulate to your benefit. When it comes to maintaining healthy levels of body fat, caloric management is at the top of that list.

Insufficient Body Fat

A far less common but more acute problem is insufficient body fat. Once you get below 3 percent for men or 12 percent for women, problems start to occur. If essential body fat gets too low, your organs can be robbed of essential cushioning, we can have trouble regulating our energy levels, and we can even have reproductive issues such as amenorrhea, which occurs in very lean female athletes. Practically, people who are too lean often feel low energy, get and stay cold easily, and have trouble recovering from exercise. Even bodybuilders only maintain the super lean body composition for the exact time that they compete and must train well above their competition numbers so they can sustain the workload it takes to build muscle.

Don't be fooled by public figures who always seem to have stable low-single-digit body fat percentages. You have no idea if they are truly healthy or what the wizard looks like behind the curtain. Here's another hint: If their skin is bright red all the time and they don't work outside, it's probably time to find somebody new. In all seriousness, people on magazine covers and in social media use cutting agents and fasting as well as lighting and filters to portray an image. Not only are many of these things false, but they are unsustainable and unhealthy. For people who are more vulnerable, exposure to these fads can perpetuate eating disorders like anorexia and bulimia, which are directly connected to anxiety issues. Body dysmorphia tends to be more common in young women but can occur in anyone regardless of gender and may require professional mental health intervention to overcome. If you are struggling with this issue, please seek help.

Muscle Mass

"Stronger people are harder to kill. And are just more useful in general."

—Coach Mark Rippetoe

The other side of the body composition coin is muscle mass. Having a healthy range of body fat is important, but so is maintaining the muscle that powers your body for everything from the tasks of daily life to rigorous exercise, if you choose to do it.

Body composition isn't just about maintaining a healthy range of body fat. Equally important is having strong, healthy muscle tissue. Sarcopenia, or age-related muscle loss, is a normal part of staying alive for a long time. Doesn't seem like much of a reward for staying alive, does it? Not only does skeletal muscle offer the more obvious physical benefits of being able to move around the world with more strength and vigor, but it also yields new and surprising benefits to our biochemistry that are important if we want to

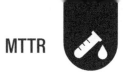

feel and perform our best for the long haul. While it is normal to see muscle mass steadily decline with age, working hard to keep as much as possible is a Sisyphean burden worth pursuing.

A friend and jiu-jitsu training partner of mine had his life saved by muscle. A lifelong weightlifter and nutrition nerd, he was hit by a car while quite literally standing around minding his own business. He was crushed between the open car door he was positioned behind and the door frame of his car. On his long road to recovery, every doctor, nurse, and physical therapist reported to him that had he not had so much muscle on his frame, he likely would have died on the spot, and the reservoir of strength he had built up accelerated his healing process.

Dr. Gabrielle Lyon calls muscle our "health insurance policy." Muscles aren't just for moving bones and looking good naked, although maintaining muscle mass certainly helps us do so. The red meat on our bodies also serves as a cushion against impact, like it did for my jiu-jitsu buddy. Muscle helps us regulate blood sugar, too. It's not as good as having a healthy pancreas that secretes insulin, but one of the recommended treatments for both type 1 diabetes (that's the genetic kind) and type 2 diabetes is increasing muscle mass. Muscle tissue is metabolically active and raises our resting metabolic rate, meaning it uses more energy simply by existing. Additionally, when muscles contract, they release special cells called myokines. Myokines are signaling molecules that not only help regulate blood sugar but also have important regulatory effects on inflammation; in fact, this may account for the positive impact that exercise has in the prevention of rheumatoid arthritis. These special cells are still in the early stages of being researched, and we have much more to learn. They show great promise, however, in helping to explain many of the benefits of resistance training on the preservation of not only physical robustness but also how the regulation of energy balance influences other aspects of performance longevity, such as Alzheimer's and dementia.

It is important to note here that while the preservation of muscle tissue is important for everybody, it is especially important for women. Women tend to be more vulnerable to muscle loss as a part of the aging process and so may need to be extra vigilant when it comes to maintaining healthy muscle tissue.

Muscle mass is often a surrogate for the maintenance of strength. Strength is a necessity. The development and maintenance of strength (and therefore muscle mass) through purposeful training is one of the most important physical gifts you can give to yourself. That statement is certainly biased to my personal experience but is corroborated by an avalanche of scientific consensus as well as by every friend, neighbor, and coworker who's ever needed help moving. Not to mention the countless people I've helped get stronger over the course of my career. When people get stronger, their bodies work better, they feel better about themselves, they develop higher levels of self-respect and confidence, and they learn to work through short-term physical discomfort in order to achieve longer-term goals. Physical strength doesn't always beget emotional strength, but the path toward the former can lead to the latter.

For a long time, building muscle and strength was associated with extreme representations like bodybuilders and powerlifters. For some, this may have presented a turnoff to building muscle and getting strong. Just like there are lots of flavors of nutritional preference to choose from, there are many ways to build muscle and stay strong. While lifting weights is the most efficient and effective way to gain strength and muscle, there's a muscle-building activity for everybody, whether it's bodyweight calisthenics, barbells, kettlebells, Pilates, or jiu-jitsu class. At the end of the day, what matters is that you do something that keeps you on the path toward strength. Is there a point where a person can have too much muscle and it can become a burden on the system? Maybe. But the truth is, even the fittest among us are far from that problem. Only at peak levels of professional bodybuilding do we see muscle as a hindrance, and even then it's hard to parse it from other habits that confound the potentially negative effects of having "excessive" muscle mass.

Maintenance of body composition isn't about seeing every muscle fiber of your butt cheeks when you wear your Speedo to the beach. It's about sustaining important metabolic and endocrine functions. Using body composition as an indicator for health doesn't have to become an obsession with percentage points. Often, the mere mental prioritization of nutrition and exercise spring forth other associated positive health habits. It can be part of a path that orients your awareness and your behavior on an anchor point that drives attention toward a more active relationship in the preservation of your health.

While the maintenance of body composition and strength is a long-term project, there are some personal health experiments in that section of the book that can help you set the stage for longer-term progress. I'll also provide some trusted resources not based on fads, gimmicks, or overwhelming information to help you engage in the longer-term experiment.

What Are You Made Of?
Indicators for Body Composition

So we've brought clarity to problems and identified our target—maintaining a healthy quality and quantity of muscle mass. So how do we measure it? First, we don't actually have a great way to specifically measure muscle mass. At present, there is no clear scientific consensus on a method of measuring muscle mass with precision. However, there are measurement devices through which reasonable inferences can be made, and those devices and methods vary in sophistication.

The most widely used and accepted method for measuring body composition is the DEXA (Dual Energy X-ray Absorptiometry). DEXA scans use X-rays to evaluate lean mass and body fat densities based on total body weight and tissue densities. DEXA readouts then differentiate the ratio of lean mass (viscera, bones, and muscle) to body fat based on that information. To date, this is the most accurate means of measurement of body composition out there, and you should be able to find one easily with a quick Google search of your area. It's relatively cheap and isn't time-consuming or difficult. You lie on a table motionless while a scanner passes over your body for about five minutes. Then a technician reads you your chart. Simple business. If you want the most valid test for body composition you can get, this is it.

Next is hydrostatic weighing. Also known as densitometry, it involves sitting on a scale while submerged in water. A technician then compares your body weight in water to your weight on land. This measurement tool derives its reading based on the differing densities of lean mass and body fat and then compares them to produce a very reliable measurement of body composition. Hydrostatic weighing is often used for athletes in university and high-performance settings but is often made available to the general public for a fee. Check with your local university's exercise physiology program. Lower rates may be available if you're willing to get measured by undergrad students attending the university.

A less precise but more accessible way to get measured is through bioelectrical impedance analysis. This measurement involves sending a small electrical signal through the body. Fat resists the signal more than lean tissue, so the rate of signal return offers insight into how much fat and how much lean tissue a person is carrying. Companies like InBody use this type of measurement in fitness studios all over the United States. Though not as precise as DEXA or hydrostatic weighing, scales and equipment like this can be helpful to track trends if used regularly enough, especially if you occasionally calibrate the reading with something more precise.

Body composition is more than just a number on the scale—it's the essence of what you're made of. Both the quality and the quantity of this composition have a profound and lasting impact on performance and longevity. Strive to improve and maintain both with unwavering consistency.

As a brief side note on measuring body composition, other options, while far more subjective, are to pay attention to how your clothes fit and how you look in pictures over time. If you have specific body composition goals, it can be helpful to take regular pictures of yourself to catalog the changes that occur. This isn't the right answer for everybody, but it can be helpful under the right circumstances.

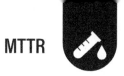

Tools: Changing Body Composition

Besides what the used-car sales teams of the fitness world will tell you, maintaining lean muscle mass and a healthy body composition is relatively straightforward as far as the science is concerned. There are a few ingredients that seem to reliably get results. Most of the arguments about this stuff are in the minutiae. The human palate is only made up of sweet, salty, sour, bitter, and umami. The vast array of culinary expressions that are displayed in cooking are influenced by tradition, culture, ingredient availability, and individual taste preferences. So too it is with maintaining a healthy body composition. In spite of what the YouTube infomercials tell you, the essentials of body composition, scientifically speaking, are pretty straightforward. It's the application where things get fun—or not so fun, depending on how you look at it.

Human biology is very complex, but let's look at a simple analogy that will help us get moving in the right direction. Imagine you're turning in a budget report at the end of the fiscal year. Before you send it up the chain, you notice that your department spent $10,000 less this year than last year. If the higher-ups in accounting see this trend, they are going to take a machete to next year's budget. If you're not using it, you probably don't need it, right? In an effort to keep your budget square, you find the most overpriced copier on the market and throw in an espresso maker for good measure. Now, when you turn in the budget, you've shown that you actually need all of the money that you were allotted. Your body treats muscles in a similar fashion. Muscles are expensive. They require lots of energy to grow and maintain. Long term, they are massively beneficial for the reasons already discussed, but they are expensive nonetheless. That's why if you stop resistance training, they go away much faster than it took you to grow them in the first place.

In short, use it or lose it.

With that said, using it does not—and I would even argue, should not—need to be complicated. Many roads lead to Rome. If you first clarify your problem and identify your target (Dashboard Function #1 again!) as specifically as possible, then it will be far easier to figure out what works best for you. Most recommendations for maintaining muscle mass come from people who are already invested in the process and, without realizing it, already have the logistical components and habits built in. One thing that can help cut through all that is to get to the heart of the thing that builds muscle mass: tension.

The primary purpose of muscles is to generate tension. They use various forms of metabolic energy to create tension between sections of bone that gets distributed through connective tissue and transmitted throughout the body to generate motion. While that may seem obvious at first glance, the lack of that consideration creates a lot of confusion and argument when it comes to which approach to use to keep muscles on your body. Some tools and methods are more efficient and effective than others, but even then, much of it boils down to the conditions under which you apply those things.

Let's take a look at a few examples.

- **Calisthenics/body weight:** Calisthenics are simply bodyweight exercises. The difficulty of these exercises can range from doing push-ups with your hands elevated on the arm of a couch all the way to performing gymnastics-type exercises like handstand walking or one-legged squatting (commonly referred to as a pistol squat). The primary way that bodyweight exercises stimulate muscle growth is through the force needed to fight against leverage. This is true for both isometric exercises (these are performed statically with no change in joint angles—think a plank exercise) and non-isometric movements. An additional way to create the appropriate stress for muscles is through the use of time under tension. A simple push-up can be made much harder by slowing it way down and keeping those tissues under tension for longer periods or by speeding it up to be as explosive as possible.

- **Kettlebells and dumbbells:** I love nearly all forms of exercise, but if I was stranded on a desert island and could have only one piece of

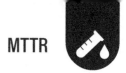

exercise equipment for the rest of my life, I would choose a kettlebell. The versatility and effectiveness of the exercises that can be performed with this handle-equipped cannonball are staggering. I keep one in my kitchen to remind me not to make excuses and get weak. Dumbbells are another great option for staying strong. Not only do they offer a wide range of exercises, but they also store away easily if you're working with limited space. There are quite literally thousands of books, videos, and articles on how to use dumbbells. Don't be perfect; be consistent. If you're not sure exactly how to meet your needs, seek help! Like bodyweight exercises, even a short supply of kettlebell or dumbbell exercises can be progressed over time using leverage (how close or far away the weight is from the fulcrum it's moving on) and tempo.

- **Barbells:** Bang for your buck in strength and muscle, barbells are king. The ergonomic shape of the bar makes it easier to symmetrically load the body with higher weights, creating more intense resistance. Movements like the deadlift and squat have been used to help accelerate and more easily measure improvements in strength for a century or more. Weightlifters, bodybuilders, and athletes use a range of barbell exercise variations to measure and develop strength, power, and muscle.

Unless you are training for a specific aesthetic or performance outcome, you can pretty much pick your flavor of resistance training. Any of these common approaches can be used as part of a plan to sustain a healthy body composition. The key is consistent application and vigorous effort. How will you know if the exercise style you've chosen has helped you alter your body composition? You measure it. More on that in the workbook.

The most important ingredient is regular and titrated exposure to overloads of force and the resulting tension. This can be done with bodyweight exercises like push-ups, pull-ups, and lunges or with external loads like barbells, dumbbells, and kettlebells. If you're looking to stay fit enough to perform well at most life tasks, then almost any combination of these exercises performed with enough consistency and effort over time will keep you in the game.

If, on the other hand, you are an athlete or another type of person with specific performance outcomes in mind, you may need to take more consideration regarding what approach you use. To that end, it's probably more about what gets the most efficient outcome in performance without robbing you of the energy required to do the thing that matters most. For example, if you're a firefighter, all of the training you do should have a positive effect on your ability to do that job for the longest time possible. There are about a million and a half ways to accomplish that as far as exercise selection goes, but what's important is that regardless of your specific taste in exercise, you clearly identify the outcome you want at a particular time, measure the effect of your selection, and then match that against the outcome you chose. Are you sensing a theme here?

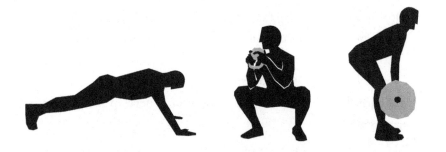

One specific note I have in regard to using various exercise methods to stay strong and maintain muscle mass is that if you decide to pursue resistance training as a beginner, it can be helpful to have some guidance on how to execute the exercises with the appropriate intention and intensity. What seems to matter most regardless of the form of resistance training is the need for consistent and deliberate physical effort.

Eating for Muscle Mass and Body Composition

Making your muscles do work is only half of the equation when it comes to building and maintaining healthy, strong muscles. The other half is

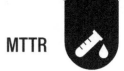
adequate caloric intake, especially protein. More and more research is showing that adequate protein intake can help with the maintenance of muscle mass, especially as we age. It also contributes to behavioral cues like satiety, the signal that you have eaten adequate food. There has been lots of conflicting information on protein over the years that has served to confuse people. Everything from protein being the boogieman all the way to a panacea has been plastered all over magazines, news articles, and social media. As usual, the truth lies somewhere in between. While there does seem to be some room in regard to how you slice up your protein intake, there are some fundamental components to getting it right. The rule of thumb for daily protein intake is 1 gram per kilogram of body weight, although women and anybody in their fifties or beyond who wants to maintain or build muscle mass may require more. Research points to whey protein as one of the best sources of protein overall, but there are plenty of plant-based options on the market that allow for adequate intake, too. Don't get lost in minutiae. Read the through line and build on that.

Performing Personal Experiments

Let's zoom out again for a moment and reconnect to the bigger picture. The most important thing when it comes to all of this is not to find a magical protocol that will deliver the results you need ad infinitum. Instead, start with a clear goal. If you need help defining that goal, get it. (Bring clarity to problems and identify targets—Dashboard Function #1). Find a way to reliably and consistently measure your progress toward that target (KPIs). Then chart a course toward that goal. In other words, run an experiment.

To that end, there are experiments in the workbook that can help you do just that.

Aerobic Health

Third on the list of surrogate markers for MTTR is aerobic health. The ability to bring in oxygen and deliver it to the tissues of your body isn't just crucial for staying alive in the most urgent sense. It also allows your tissues to heal effectively, which has widespread effects on performance longevity. Perhaps most importantly, aerobic health has a powerful effect on your ability to use energy efficiently. The maintenance of aerobic health isn't just about being able to run a marathon; it's about reducing the total stress load on your heart and lungs as they do their job of delivering vital oxygen to the rest of your body. I hope that sounds as important as it is.

The importance of developing and maintaining cardiorespiratory fitness has long been known and is what inspired the running craze of the 1970s (a photo of Farrah Fawcett and Lee Majors out for a jog appeared on the cover of *People* in 1977). Increased aerobic capacity has been shown to do everything from improve performance on high-intensity sprint recovery in athletes to help prevent chronic diseases like Alzheimer's and dementia. Not only that, but aerobic exercise is also critical in the maintenance of blood markers like hemoglobin A1C, an indicator of insulin sensitivity and prediabetes, and HDL, the "good cholesterol." In fact, aerobic capacity has been shown to have inverse relationships with nearly every known marker of mortality.

To some degree, it's intuitive that cardiorespiratory function is essential for health and performance. The talking heads of health tell us over and over that it is. But what does aerobic health and function really mean? What does maintaining it really do for us in terms of shorter-term performance but also as a leading indicator of longevity?

Sheer Energy

Let's break things down a bit more. What we are talking about here is your body's ability to bring in air from the environment, pull oxygen from it (air is only about 21 percent oxygen), and then deliver that oxygen from the pulmonary system (the lungs) into circulation, where it will be pumped through your bloodstream to tissues that use oxygen to generate energy. The keyword there (and really in all of health) is energy. The fundamental idea behind all of this is that you want your body to efficiently and effectively

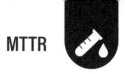

generate energy so that you can do the work of life and performance. Keep that goal in mind as we continue deeper into nerdery.

While the way the body creates and uses energy is vastly more complex than I have space for here (many textbooks are devoted to such study), the CliffsNotes version should suffice for our purposes. The human body uses three primary pathways to create energy: the phosphocreatine, the glycolytic, and the aerobic. The first two produce energy without oxygen, while the third, the aerobic, uses oxygen as its primary fuel. Without diving too deeply into energy system physiology, I'll provide a short description of each, as later it will help us imbue the special significance of aerobic function in particular.

Let's look at the two anaerobic pathways to energy first. The phosphocreatine pathway is only effective for about five seconds and does not use oxygen as part of its process of creating energy, making it anaerobic. By its very nature, this energy system is not equipped to sustain any continuous activity. It's high octane but low duration.

Also anaerobic is the glycolytic system. This system produces energy through the use of carbohydrates stored as glycogen in muscle cells. The glycolytic system produces pyruvate and lactate as by-products of the energy-making process, which can build up with time and work. The glycolytic system is also a higher-octane energy producer, but because its fuel source is more available, it can produce energy for much longer, for around three minutes. While technically anaerobic in its production of energy, the glycolytic system uses oxygen to convert these by-products present from the chemical process into new glycolytic energy. Being efficient at getting oxygen into the body and downstream to muscles then is important even if oxygen is not the primary fuel. When you can't feed enough oxygen into the system to maintain the rate of work, you can reach acidosis, and muscles begin to contract at lower and lower rates, essentially slowing down your ability to perform work and increasing your need to rest so the system can in effect reset. Both anaerobic systems are important to overall function (otherwise we would not have them) but are more costly in terms of how reliably they can continue to produce energy.

Now we have the star of the show. The aerobic system is the most pervasive supplier of energy in the body because oxygen is the most readily available fuel source. Aerobic energy is produced by using oxygen to break down carbohydrates and fatty acids. When the body produces energy aerobically, the process is much slower, but it is far more sustainable. While anaerobic systems last seconds to minutes, the aerobic system can continue to produce energy for hours. You may have guessed that the aerobic system is the primary way that the body produces energy for all basic functions. It isn't just about low- to moderate-intensity exercise; the aerobic energy pathway delivers oxygen so you can maintain rudimentary life functions. The delivery of oxygen to the body is dependent on how well your lungs function, the power and efficiency of your heart, and the health of the circulatory system. These three factors work together to ensure that oxygen gets to where it needs to go so that sustainable energy can be created for the body and brain.

Speaking technically, you are never entirely in one or another of these energy systems. They are operating in varying percentages of your total energy production based on what you are doing and your baseline levels of fitness and genetics. Some muscles can be working primarily aerobically while others are in an anaerobic state. In other words, when we say somebody is anaerobic or aerobic, we are referring to the source of net percentage of energy expenditure. The human body is agnostic when it comes to energy production and will get good at using whatever you condition it to (even if that is a *lack* of conditioning). What differs is the availability of the fuel that runs each of these systems and the cost associated with running them.

With that said, the aerobic system is by far the most energy efficient and remains an essential focus even if you don't want to run the Boston Marathon or cycle in the Tour de France. Even in sports that are primarily anaerobically based, like wrestling and weightlifting, the effective delivery of oxygen ensures that athletes can repeat bouts of high effort and their bodies can heal effectively from the stress of training and competition. They may not require the same levels of aerobic performance as highly specialized endurance athletes, but a powerful and efficient aerobic system never made anybody perform worse.

Let's look at an example of how these energy systems work practically.

Imagine you're on a bike ride with your best friend to meet a third friend for coffee. The coffee shop is about five miles away, with a few changes in terrain along the way. You ride this route daily as part of your routine, but your best friend has been mostly sedentary for the last five years and hasn't ridden a bike in nearly that long.

As you set off, you maintain a relaxed pace—about ten to twelve miles per hour on flat pavement. For you, this is entirely aerobic; your heart rate is low, and you can easily chat. Your friend, on the other hand, is keeping up but breathing harder, and you notice their sentences getting shorter. They're already working closer to their aerobic threshold, where their body starts relying more on anaerobic metabolism to keep up.

Then you realize you're running late and pick up the pace to around sixteen miles per hour. You still feel in control, though talking requires slightly more effort. Your friend, however, has fallen behind. When you call out that a traffic light is coming up, they can only muster a wave. At this point, your aerobic system is still dominant, efficiently fueling your effort, but your friend is increasingly tapping into anaerobic glycolysis—a more demanding energy system that burns through carbohydrates faster and generates metabolic by-products like lactate.

As the light turns yellow, you decide to sprint through. For these few seconds, you're using the phosphocreatine system, which provides rapid energy for explosive efforts of under fifteen seconds. You clear the intersection and look back, seeing that your friend only had enough left in the tank to reach the median. They give you a thumbs-up, but they're visibly out of breath. As you slow down to recover, your heart rate quickly returns to baseline, thanks to your well-trained aerobic system. When your friend catches up, they're still struggling to talk, taking longer to bring their heart rate and breathing under control.

You're almost at the coffee shop, but first, you have to cross a steep bridge. You push into the pedals, maintaining a steady power output. This effort still leans on your aerobic system, but now anaerobic glycolysis is kicking in to provide additional fuel, causing a mild burn in your legs. Your friend, however, doesn't make it all the way up—they dismount about half-way and start pushing their bike. The increasing energy demand has caught up with them.

By the time your friend reaches the top, they're heavily fatigued, drenched in sweat, and needing a longer break. After nearly ten minutes, you both coast down the other side toward the coffee shop. As you park your bikes and place your orders, you feel back to normal, fully recovered. Your friend, on the other hand, is still breathing heavily, likely still burning a higher percentage of carbohydrates compared to your more efficient reliance on fat oxidation from aerobic conditioning.

This ride illustrates an important point: *Your body's ability to efficiently generate and use energy is a key marker of health and performance.* The more aerobically fit you are, the more effectively you recover between efforts, delay fatigue, and rely on sustainable energy sources. Conversely, when someone is deconditioned—or dealing with metabolic, cardiovascular, or pulmonary disease—their body struggles to supply oxygen efficiently, making even moderate activity feel disproportionately hard. Over time, these inefficiencies place stress on vital systems, reducing function and increasing long-term health risks.

Regardless of whether you're a competitive athlete or just someone looking to stay healthy for life, building a robust aerobic system is essential—it's what keeps you moving longer, recovering faster, and staying resilient in the face of life's physical demands.

I'll make one final point here about aerobic health and energy delivery in general. These things work on a sliding scale. Here I compared you to a friend in this story who wasn't aerobically conditioned enough to keep up with you on a bike ride, but deconditioning of these energy systems can slide all the way down to daily tasks like walking up stairs becoming what seem like physical fitness challenges. These things tend to sneak up on us until we run out of compensatory strategies. If you're not sure what to look for or don't have good systems of measurement and maintenance, health malfunctions can occur in what seems like a sudden chain of events.

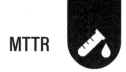

What I presented here is a dramatically simplified explanation of human energy systems but should suffice for demonstrating the vital role that oxygen plays in powering performance and sustaining health. If you want to scratch the physiology itch a bit deeper, I recommend Dr. Andy Galpin's work. He has volumes of videos and interviews online as well as a great podcast, *Perform*, where he dives deep into these topics.

Next up, let's dive into various indicators for aerobic health and how they can be used to track this vital aspect of performance longevity.

Indicators: Measuring Oxygen Delivery

Volume Oxygen Maximum (VO2 max)

VO2 max is a measurement of your maximum volume of oxygen intake in a minute reflected as milliliters per kilogram per minute (ml/kg/min). It is widely considered the gold standard of aerobic capacity, and this indicator seems to be the single most consistent metric with health span available today. To assess VO2 max, subjects (usually in a laboratory setting) wear a mask that measures gas exchange (namely oxygen and carbon dioxide) and a heart rate monitor while performing exercise at varying levels of intensity and duration. This is typically done while exercising on a treadmill or, when the utmost precision is required, a specialized stationary bike. The test usually lasts between ten and fifteen minutes, after which a laboratory technician issues a score. This score is a direct reflection of the subject's ability to perform work while the body is using oxygen as its primary fuel source.

Often, local universities will perform this test for a fee. If this option isn't available to you, there are reasonable corollary tests used in health and athletics, like the Cooper Test (a twelve-minute maximum walk or run for distance), among others. Some of these methods are referenced in the personal health experiments in the workbook and have been validated against the more precise gas exchange marker discussed here.

Resting Heart Rate (RHR)

RHR is another common metric used in the triangulation of cardiorespiratory fitness. Measured as beats per minute during the lowest activity of the day, RHR is a reliable way to gain insight into your aerobic health. If you measure it using a wearable device, your RHR will be taken overnight during deep sleep to get a true reading. If you don't have a wearable device, don't sweat it. You can still get reasonable enough information by taking your pulse when you first wake up in the morning. You can count heartbeats for an entire minute or count for fifteen seconds and then multiply by four.

A lower RHR generally indicates improved aerobic function, while a higher RHR can point to impaired aerobic function. Fluctuations from day to day don't indicate changes in your aerobic system that you should be concerned with. Like all of our metrics, be sure to watch trends over time. If your RHR is generally improving, that means your parasympathetic nervous system is responding to better conditioning. In other words, your body doesn't need to work as hard to deal with life stuff. As my friend and strength and conditioning wizard Tim Kelly says, try to "raise the floor." In other words, as you make attempts to improve, focus on making the bottom of the average improve over time so that your old best day is now your new worst day.

Heart Rate Recovery (HRR)

HRR is another valid, accessible, reliable indicator for aerobic fitness as compared to both VO2 max and RHR. HRR is one of the most accessible indicators for cardiopulmonary performance longevity and can be used by nearly anybody, anywhere. While it's not as sophisticated as VO2 max, its accessibility means you can track it more regularly to identify ranges and trends that might not be as readily available as testing that needs to be done in a performance laboratory.

To calculate HRR:

1. **Perform intense exercise.** Engage in a bout of intense exercise, such as sprinting or cycling, to elevate your heart rate significantly.

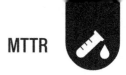

2. **Measure maximum heart rate.** At the end of the exercise, record your maximum heart rate (in beats per minute, or BPM) by using a heart rate monitor or manually checking your pulse.

3. **Set a timer.** Set a timer for 1 minute immediately after the exercise ends.

4. **Take a reading at 30 seconds.** At the 30-second mark, measure your heart rate again and note the value.

5. **Take another reading at 1 minute.** At the 1-minute mark, measure your heart rate again and note this value as well.

6. **Calculate heart rate recovery.** Subtract the heart rate at 30 seconds or 1 minute from your maximum heart rate. For example, max HR of 180 BPM – HR after 1 minute of 150 BPM = HRR of 30 BPM.

Note: A more significant drop in HR generally indicates a higher degree of cardiovascular fitness.

In the workbook, you'll use these metrics in various ways to perform personal health experiments for the aerobic system.

Tools for Better Aerobic Performance

Steady State/Zone 2 Training

Let's start with the talk of the town. Right now, Zone 2 training is the most doted-upon training method for improving VO2 max. Rightfully so. This training has been shown over and over to be an effective way to boost aerobic function and the chemistry of performance longevity. Zone 2 training is performed by exercising at an intensity that maintains your heart rate at approximately 60 to 75 percent of its max. A good rule of thumb for this range is to be working at a continuous pace for twenty to thirty minutes in which you could hold a conversation. This type of exercise keeps you in sustainable ranges of aerobic work for thirty to forty-five minutes at a time. The common recommendation for the general population is an hour and a half to two hours per week, while aerobically adapted athletes may need more. Longevity expert Dr. Peter Attia is a fantastic resource if you want to dig more deeply into this topic.

High-Intensity Interval Training (HIIT)

HIIT is another option if you want to improve VO2 max and aerobic capacity more generally. HIIT is working in short bursts at maximum effort. This style of training has been shown to have a powerful ability to improve energy system capacity but also is a massive time-saver, which makes it very attractive for most people. HIIT can be

- Short intervals of one minute or less followed by longer rest periods

- Short intervals with short rest like the infamous Tabata Interval (twenty seconds of all-out work followed by ten seconds of rest, repeated eight times)

- Longer intervals of two minutes of intense effort followed by longer periods of moderate work lasting around fifteen minutes

While all of these intervals have been associated with beneficial changes in aerobic function, the shortest intervals seem to help the least fit individuals make the most rapid changes, while longer intervals were necessary for fitter individuals and led to more significant improvements in VO2 max.

Low-Intensity Aerobic Exercise

Low-intensity aerobic exercise has been shown to improve aerobic function, but mostly in people who are already at a deficit, such as obese or sedentary individuals. Walking, for example, is an easily accessible way for a deconditioned person to introduce moderate cardiorespiratory training stress to their body in a way that is not injurious. As fitness increases, more stress will be necessary to maintain or improve aerobic fitness. It's a bummer, but alas, it is the nature of these things. With that said, adding challenges in terrain or loading the body (like a rucksack) can be a simple accessible way to increase walking intensity enough to elicit an aerobic response. The only way to know for sure is to measure and try. While low-intensity aerobic

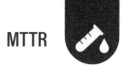

exercise may not offer a direct effect on cardiopulmonary health, it can be a way to improve health habits in general, including mental health status and sleep hygiene, both of which can affect performance longevity.

Aerobic health is a crucial part of the bigger picture when it comes to managing our biochemistry. Don't let the details dizzy your head too much. The explanations of how these things work are complex, but the solutions to managing them are simple. The great thing is that you can get as granular and sophisticated as you like—or not. What matters most is that you find a suitable way to pay attention to and measure the important aspects of your MTTR. Don't try to make things perfect or fancy. Over time, your understanding will grow, but you have to start experimenting if you want to build these skills. If you're not sure where to start, check out the workbook!

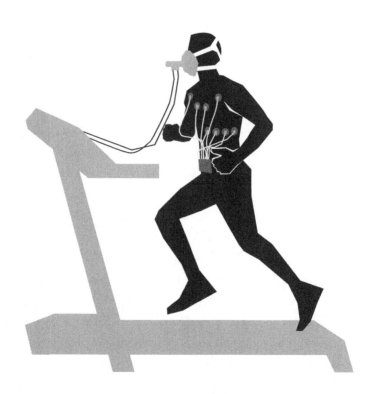

BAG O' CHEMICALS

*"Compounding interest is the eighth wonder of the world.
He who understands it, earns it—he who doesn't, pays it."*

—Albert Einstein

This isn't just true for money. It's true for health, too. While some bio-markers can be changed pretty quickly with nutritional adjustments, like vitamin D, others can only be sufficiently buffered through time and effort—strength and VO2 max, for example. If you realize later in life that you should have saved money or invested and are behind the curve, should you throw your hands up and say, "To hell with it all"? No. You should start saving today. As the old Chinese saying goes, "The best time to plant a tree was twenty years ago. The second best time is now."

The three proxy biomarkers presented in this chapter are by no means the alpha and the omega of what drives all of human biochemical function. They are, however, big levers you can pull to lift much of the load of performance longevity. There are micronutrients, enzymes, supplements, as well as many more indicators that can support performance longevity. The higher the degree of performance you want to maintain, the more precise you may need to be in your application of biochemistry to maintain it. With that said, I have worked with many elite performers who were having trouble and found themselves to be falling short in at least one of these three categories. Even the highest-achieving among us are still human.

Human beings are more than a bag of chemicals, but chemistry matters. The study and application of chemistry to the biology of human beings saves lives and has allowed us to achieve a never-before-seen level of precision in health technology. Not only that, but these technologies have been democratized so effectively that nearly anybody can order a basic health panel on their phone, march down to the lab, give blood, and get the results within a few days. Truly amazing.

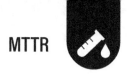

The challenge that remains is what to do with all of this information. Big data has arrived, and it is only getting bigger. It behooves us to be able to sniff out the information that is most important to us, have a plan of action that we can use to make sensible change, and then see if we made a difference in the measurement we chose. You know, science and stuff.

As access to more and more refined layers of data grows, so too can the confusion that comes with that data. (Wasn't it the Notorious B.I.G. who rapped, "Mo data, mo problems"?) Computer scientists and data analysts who work in interpretation will tell you that with a big enough data set, all data becomes statistically relevant. Which bits will you use to make critical decisions about your health?

Blood work, sleep, body composition, and aerobic health are essential indicators for your Performance Longevity Dashboard. But what is more essential than any single indicator is the ability to think critically about how all of the component parts within MIND, MVMT, and MTTR come together to form the big picture of performance longevity.

What are the key concepts for doing so? That's what the next section of this book is all about.

SECTION THREE
TUNING THE HUMAN

How does everything you've read up until now work together and develop into a sustainable lifestyle of performance longevity? In this section, I'll tie up loose ends and get to how what you've read in previous chapters is practically applied.

Section Three wraps everything up into a philosophy that guides you toward developing the skills and mindset needed for performance longevity. After zooming in close in Section Two, Section Three backs out a bit to consider the bigger picture.

These last two chapters of *Check Engine Light* examine how differences in personality can influence your approach to health and performance as well as how to develop an experimental mindset. Section Three highlights my deepest hope for you in writing this book: that you can become an autonomous and informed arbiter of your own performance longevity.

"Health is not a state; it's a practice."

—m. c. schraefel

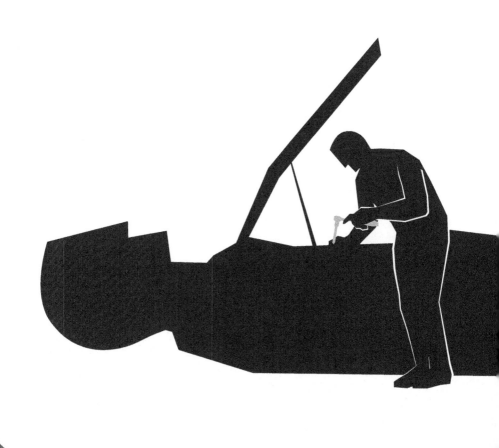

CHAPTER 7: | The Bigger Picture

L et's take a moment and come up for air from that deep dive on the M3 Model. It's important that we don't get stuck in the weeds. Remember, the purpose of the M3 Model is to make it easier to categorize the indicators that you want to put on your Performance Longevity Dashboard as well as select tools for your toolkit. Any specific indicator or tool that I share in this book is not in any way intended to serve as an end point. In fact, to think of them as such would do both them and you a disservice.

With that said, I hope you will use the indicators I've already discussed as well as the personal health experiments in the workbook as jumping-off points to learn to tread water. Some of the examples of indicators may be old hat to you, and others may be fresh insights. A real measure of success will be if you take the principles shared here to heart and develop a more discerning and critical attitude toward your performance longevity and how you want to pursue it.

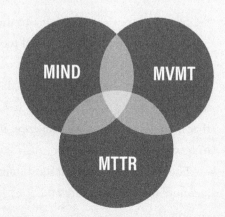

Another important reminder I want to issue here is that in reality, none of the categories MIND, MVMT, and MTTR exists independently of the others (or in truth, at all). All three are braided together. If you move the needle on one, you affect all three. For example, moving better and reducing back pain could improve the quality of your sleep and thus change your mood for the better (your significant others can send thank-you letters directly to my publisher). The magnitude of that change can vary based on what you're emphasizing, but a human being is but one integrated system. What these three categories do provide are points of discernment where you can temporarily segregate concepts and actions to gain insight. Zoom in for clarity; zoom out for understanding. Practically speaking, this is important because as you experiment, you may get unexpected results. Biology does not always organize itself according to your hypothesis. Be open to the possibility of surprising outcomes. That's when it gets really exciting!

As we move forward, we're going look at the bigger picture of performance longevity. There are subtle points of awareness that can improve your health and performance journey and prepare you to get the most value when you apply the concepts in this book.

TOOLS CAN BE INDICATORS, INDICATORS CAN BE TOOLS

You may have noticed that some of the items I talked about in Section 2 can be used as both indicators and tools. If and when you find one of those things, you've got yourself a keeper. One example could be Sun Salutation from Chapter 5. In the "Function Check" section, I talked about how Sun Salutation can be used as a litmus test for daily movement. You might find that if you practice it with diligence, it will be a way for you to gain access to new ranges of motion, too.

The overlap of tools and indicators tends to happen with practices that are more organic in nature and don't have a technological interface. It's hard to turn the indicators of blood work into tools for modulating the chemicals in your blood—not gonna happen. But tools like Morning Pages for MIND (see page 117), Sun Salutation for MVMT (see pages 180 to 182), and even food choices for MTTR (see pages 225 to 227) can serve as both tools and indicators. Food choices as indicators? Sure. Isn't there a food that you tend to crave when you want to celebrate or you feel sad? Wanting "comfort food" is an indicator for wanting, well, comfort. Pay attention to how your mind and body are connecting with your experience through the use of your tools and indicators. That's the whole game.

SPRING CLEANING: CHALLENGE AS AN AUDIT

Like most people, I'm sure you have some sort of routine for how you tackle the cleaning duties in your home. Those chores are organized not just by who is responsible but also by timing: washing the dishes every day, taking out the trash every couple of days, vacuuming the floor once a week, and changing the air filter once a month. In addition to those recurring and overlapping short-term duties, there is longer-range deep cleaning: You pull all of the pictures down, scrub the walls, and reorganize the shelves. You roll up the rugs and sweep up the crud that has built up underneath. Essentially, you perform a large-scale audit of your home. This keeps your home from getting filthy and breaking down, and in the process you might discover larger issues that need your attention before they become even bigger problems. Just as deep cleaning reveals dust and grime you didn't even know was there, structured physical or mental challenges expose the weak spots in your performance and resilience.

One of the best ways to motivate an internal audit is through a purposefully orchestrated challenge. It's easy to gloss over the deeper questions of performance longevity in your day-to-day routine, even if you already have generally good habits. Even well-intentioned routines can lead to complacency over time. Strategic stress tests highlight blind spots in your health and performance, helping you refine focus and reinforce key areas like MIND, MVMT, and MTTR. For athletes, competition provides these challenges. For those of us who don't compete in specific events, it's important to push our bodies and minds into states of work and discomfort on a regular basis to see how we respond. I don't care what your biomarkers say if you can't rise to meet the trial that life throws at you.

Using a formal challenge as a sort of spring cleaning for your body and mind can provide you with interesting types of critical feedback. It can penetrate surface layers of information to expose a deeper truth about where you really stand. Let me give you an example from my own experience.

I got COVID-19 for the first time in late 2020. I went down hard. It was like the flu from hell. I was quarantined on my couch for four or five days in a pile of blankets and sweat. Luckily, it didn't advance to a more serious cardiorespiratory issue like it did for scores of others. After the five-day kick in the butt, I started to come through and felt pretty good when doing normal stuff around the house—piddling, light chores, walking my dogs. I thought I was good to go. A week to the day after I got sick, I needed to find out where I really stood—not just how I felt while walking around the house, but whether my body could handle real work again. That's why I picked up the kettlebell that lives in my kitchen (yes, I really do keep a kettlebell in my kitchen) and put myself through a small, controlled stress test. I've been swinging this kettlebell for a very long time, so I was used to the weight, and I was in good shape before getting sick, so I had no reason to believe it would present a novel challenge, but I wanted a deeper look into how my body would handle the increased workload. About seven repetitions in, my heart rate skyrocketed. I stopped swinging the kettlebell immediately and thought, "I guess I'm not as well as I thought."

This little wakeup call accomplished two things. Without it, I might have assumed I was fully recovered and jumped back into my normal routine too soon, risking a more serious setback. More importantly, it reminded me that objective self-assessments often reveal things that subjective feelings miss (see Section One of this book). This is the exact purpose of structured challenges: to expose blind spots before they cause bigger problems. First, it let me know that my physiology wasn't nearly as recovered as I assumed it was, and I might need to temper my activity for a couple more days. Second, I got a clue into what to expect if circumstances required me to forcefully exert myself. This might not seem like a big deal on face value, but lots of people "pull their backs" and get hernias not because they didn't lift with their legs like the IKEA box told them to, but because they didn't have an accurate assessment of their true capacity to begin with.

This is the other purpose that planned challenges serve: They provide a reality check, revealing how you'll actually respond when stress hits. If you only rely on how you "think" you'll perform, you risk getting caught off-guard when it matters most. This applies not just to recovery from illness but to long-term resilience and performance as well. By regularly exposing yourself to controlled stressors, you can refine your ability to handle them, making you more robust over time. Being healthy and performing well isn't just about numbers on a page or checking boxes so you can live longer. It's about knowing you can act when it matters most. The question is, how do you know? Just like my post-COVID kettlebell swings served as a personal audit, you need ways to periodically check where you truly stand.

That's where structured challenges come in.

What do these challenges look like, exactly? You can do mini-audits or larger-scale challenges that require more planning. They both have their place, and doing them can help you stay attuned to both your strengths and your shortcomings.

Let's start with smaller challenges. These are usually in the form of unobtrusive daily check-ins that are performed over a relatively short timeline. For example, every winter I do a kettlebell swing challenge. I do 100 swings, first thing every day, for 100 consecutive days. I can break them up into however many sets I want to; I just have to get them done. These swings do not take the place of other exercise I'm doing. That's not the role they play for me. Instead, it's about doing something first thing in the morning that I really don't want to do. By about the sixtieth day, which is usually in February, it is still very dark when I wake up. This is when I find out whether I'll stick with my commitment. I could stop and nobody would ever know. Do I have the discipline to keep going? This mini-audit by kettlebell isn't an indicator of fitness for me. Instead, what I learn is how I react internally to another day of monotonous kettlebell swinging while my eyelids are still ungluing.

A couple more important points about creating audits for MIND, MVMT, and MTTR:

Plan it. Planning is the key when it comes to regularly stepping into challenges. Improper planning can also provide a convenient "out." Here are a few steps that can help:

- Decide what the challenge is. Make it an actual challenge.

- Say it out loud to at least two or three people who care enough about you to hold you accountable.

- Plan a time and date(s) when this challenge will occur.

- Stick to it. That's actually part of the challenge.

Choose real challenges. Misunderstanding around this topic is common—what's routine for you isn't a challenge. A true challenge involves friction, whether it is internal resistance ("This is hard, I don't feel like it") or an external test of your physical ability.

- What am I avoiding?

- What don't I want to do?

- What causes internal friction for me?

- Where do I really need to grow?

It is the weak point in the dam that will crack when the river rises. Give yourself to the challenges. Some of us know how to lean into being physically uncomfortable, so intense exercise looks challenging from the outside but may not be where the most growth is available. For me personally, I can do physical work ad nauseam. So, while physical challenges are hard, it was much more of a challenge for me to learn to control my temper. At the end of the day, only you know whether something is truly challenging you or not. If you decide to take the easy route, when you bump into true audits of your capacity, you will not have the skills to navigate them.

As with most everything else, the scale is a sliding one. I don't expect my grandmother to devise the same personal challenges as a thirty-year-old firefighter would. The most important thing is to orient yourself toward challenges that show you what is working and what needs additional attention. For my grandma, it might be going up and down the stairs from the basement to the attic. If she can do that, she knows she's in good shape. If she struggles, she knows she has to kick it up a gear and take walks more frequently. For the firefighter, it might be the obstacle course at the training center. In either case, you don't want to wait until the moment you're broke to do an audit.

SELF-REFLECTION QUESTIONS

What purposeful challenge have you engaged in recently?

_____

_____

What did you learn? Give specific examples from MIND, MVMT, and/or MTTR.

_____

_____

YOUR HEALTH GPA

Managing health is like a GPA	
B– for 20 years	A+ for one day
~~ B–	~~~~~~~~~~~ A+
~~ B–	~~~~~~~~~~~ F
~~ B–	~~~~~~~~~~~ F
~~ B–	~~~~~~~~~~~ F
~~ B–	~~~~~~~~~~~ F
GPA: 2.7	**GPA: 0.6**

As you pay closer attention to your indicator lights, you start to realize all of the things you've been missing and all of the things you need to do to keep this machine of yours running. This onslaught of information can be overwhelming, to say the least. Go to bed on time, limit bright lights at night, stretch before bed, eat whole foods but not too much, do Sun Salutation, go for walks, shut off your phone, be in touch with your emotions, keep your relationships in check—the list goes on and on. How in the heck can you manage to corral all of these needs to achieve performance longevity? Well, you can't. At least not all at once with the wave of a magic wand.

Rather than think of performance longevity as a single state of being, think of it as a distribution of points on a scoreboard. Imagine there are 150 points you can measure and implement to get a perfect performance longevity score (and that number is made up, so don't worry about it). Those points are divided equally between the three categories of MIND, MVMT, and MTTR, each with 50 points. If you did half of all of the things you could do in each category, that would add up to 25 points each, or a total score of 75 points. That's 50 percent. It might not sound like a lot, but what if you started at 30 points? Or 10? Then an increase to 75 points would be pretty darn awesome, and that's what matters most: long-term improvement.

I can stretch this analogy out a little further. The 25 points you start with in each category won't necessarily remain evenly distributed. For example, you might earn all 50 possible points in MVMT but only 10 in MTTR and 15 in MIND. Maybe your diet slips and you lose some points there, but you make improvements in your exercise routine and gain points in that category. A little bit of variation in how the points are distributed is normal. What you don't want are huge drops in your total score that reflect a net loss in performance longevity.

It's also essential to cultivate an awareness of the fact that life may reduce your points in certain columns in spite of your best efforts. If you have a new baby, for example, sleep (which falls under MTTR) is going to take a hit. If you slip on the ice and break your ankle, MVMT is likely to suffer. What then? Don't sweat it. Buffer the other areas as best you can and formulate a plan for rebuilding in your weakened category. Disruptions in daily rhythms are a normal part of the larger rhythm of life. Find indicators and tools that help you keep your total score as high as possible and stick with them. Those are likely your proximal tools!

Another simple way to think of the net effect of all of this is like building your health GPA. In school, your grade point average is a collection of small behaviors that accumulate over time. Homework, quizzes, projects, written papers, and exams add up to determine your academic score. This doesn't happen all at once but over years of school. Some subjects come more naturally, and with others you might struggle. Sometimes you study with discipline, and other times you might slack off a bit. There can be bumps in the road you can't do anything about, too. Factors like time missed for being sick, very strict teachers, inadequate support at home or at school, and more have influence over your grades as you progress through your academic career.

If you think back on your academic history, it's not straight lines up and down. It's a bumpy road that culminates in the net outcome of your

GPA. Maybe one semester you got two A's, two B's, and two C's. That's a B average. Next semester you got all B's—your C's went up but your A's went down. Still a B average. Just like the grades on your academic report card, the grades on your performance longevity report card will move, too. While it is important to give the individual "subjects" that you manage in MIND, MVMT, and MTTR their due attention, remember to zoom back out and stay focused on the bigger picture of your health GPA.

SELF-REFLECTION QUESTIONS

If you had a performance longevity report card, what would your GPA be?

_____

_____

What fluctuations occur in different "classes" during a year, for example? Think about how things like sleep, exercise, and mental health go up and down.

_____

_____

What aspects of those could be improved to raise your GPA?

_____

_____

What things are you already doing well that you could do extra credit in to buffer the things you're not so good at?

_____

_____

ZOOM IN, ZOOM OUT

You may have noticed that throughout this book, I repeat a phrase over and over: Zoom in for clarity; zoom out for understanding. These two lenses offer complementary views of the same reality. When we zoom in, we see details. Zooming in gives us measurables and values. The close view provides precision and helps us clarify what exactly we are looking at. A microscope is great for looking at the cellular structure of a leaf, but it's not a good tool if you want to understand weather patterns. Conversely, studying satellite images may not be your best bet if you want to learn about photosynthesis. They both have their place in understanding the full picture of life on our planet, and they should be used together to comprehend the larger picture.

Similarly, we now have wearables that can give us detailed information about things like our heart rate, sleep cycles, and body temperature. This data can be useful in managing aspects of our health and performance with added precision. They do not, however, speak to the larger context in which these measurements are occurring. Your Apple Watch doesn't know whether you were stressed this Wednesday because you were partying on vacation or because you hit a new personal record on your deadlift—it just knows you were stressed.

It can become necessary to enhance the resolution on single parts of the whole performance longevity picture—to zoom in. For example, not too long ago I was traveling quite a bit for work and started feeling a little sluggish in some of my regular exercises, so I decided to weigh in and get my body composition measured. I'd gained thirteen pounds since the previous year's check-in, and ten of those pounds were abdominal fat. (Apparently, there is a tipping point to dark chocolate–covered almonds. Who knew?) I'm over six feet tall and weigh well over two hundred pounds, so visually I'd barely noticed a difference, but it wasn't a trend I wanted to accept. The lag in my pull-ups is what set off the warning bell that made me zoom in to calibrate my sense of what was happening with a more granular measurement. I stayed zoomed in and reduced my caloric intake using the nutrition app Carbon, which kept me honest about exactly how many calories I was putting into my body. Focusing in on details allowed for a higher degree of precision while I was working toward a specific change and measuring the results. This same idea can be applied to tracking your sleep or writing in a journal to audit your thinking.

As important as zooming in is, the details do not represent the full picture. Looking closely at measurables is essential for precision, but it doesn't tell you the relevance of the things you are measuring. It'd be like a police sniper getting a perfect headshot…on the hostage. High accuracy, wrong target. That's why it's important to zoom out as well—to make sure that the metrics and data you are putting together are serving the big picture of what you are trying to accomplish. Many of us are prone to these kinds of errors because we fixate on single points of change as the keys to the castle.

I saw the failure to zoom out cause trouble back when my wife, Thomi, and I were still running CrossFit Virginia Beach. One of the benefits of being part of a CrossFit gym is that software is often deployed to help people keep track of their workouts. The exercises, sets, and repetitions as well as any personal records achieved are displayed for both individuals and the community. The upside of communal scorekeeping is that clients feel pressure to give their best effort. The downside is that clients would forget about context as a relevant factor in their progress. Everybody likes to see measurable progress, but our clients were not professional weightlifters. They were people lifting weights as part of a comprehensive plan to be healthier. When clients would zoom in too much on the details of the exact poundages they lifted or the exercise times they set from day to day, we would remind them of the bigger picture of why they were there and how much total progress they had made over a longer timeline. Improving and even "maintaining" health are not linear trajectories. There are ups and downs, gains and setbacks. Even the larger context of life outside the gym makes a difference in the story that the metrics tell. Zooming out can help you make sure that the things you are measuring remain relevant to the big picture so that you don't sink the ship just because you get blown off course.

It's important not to get stranded in the clouds, either. Staying up there can cause you to miss critical details in your indicators that not only let you off the hook when you shouldn't be, but also rob you of the opportunity to measure real progress. *Squeaky brakes? I don't need to get my brakes checked; I can stop just fine.* Until one day you drive through a puddle and now you can't stop at all. If you never take a look at the coarse metrics that drive your health, the outcomes can seem shrouded in mystery, or you can make assumptions that lead you astray. In controlled weight loss studies, people who have never tracked their caloric intake underestimate their daily intake by around 1,000 calories. If you're getting a health result you don't want, being imprecise can make it harder to know what to change in order to correct it. If you're getting one you do want, it's hard to know which actions to repeat in order to sustain it. Health then becomes a game of press and guess. This happens quite a bit, and it's why you need indicators on a dashboard in the first place.

Zooming in gives you access to detailed information that can easily be measured and tracked to reflect outcomes. Zooming out ensures that the information you are getting is relevant to the big picture. Zoom in for clarity, zoom out for understanding. Interestingly, there are people who seem to get stuck in either zooming in or zooming out and have some predictable advantages and challenges with how they organize their approach to health. The performance longevity avatars described next offer a continuum that makes it easier to spot when and where you are getting stuck on this sliding scale.

SELF-REFLECTION QUESTIONS

These examples you provide here don't necessarily have to be related to health and performance. Think of examples from any aspect of life, and then bring it back to performance longevity.

Name a time when getting more detailed (zooming in) helped you. This could be achieving a goal, changing a habit, or solving a problem.

_____

_____

Name a time when getting stuck in the details may have hindered you.

_____

_____

Conversely, name a time where not knowing the details (zooming out) helped you.

_____

_____

What's an example of a time when not knowing the details hindered you?

_____

_____

THE AVATARS: ENGINEERS AND INTUITIVES

An important lesson I've learned as a human performance professional is that people are different. Individual differences and responses count when you're trying to influence human behavior. It doesn't matter what the most thorough research study in the world says if the way that information is presented doesn't jibe with a particular person's personality. We all have our preferences and peccadilloes, and those things affect the way we see the world and therefore how we manage and respond to health information. Understanding where you are on the continuum of viewpoints can help guard against fallacies that come when you start to analyze your indicators and choose your tools. To help you find where you fall on that spectrum, I've identified two avatars in the realm of performance longevity: the Engineer and the Intuitive.

Engineers like facts, figures, and data. Their conscientious nature makes them detail oriented and disciplined. Engineers want to know about the plans and the evidence. When Engineers use wearable devices, they pay attention to the feedback. They know their steps for the day and the week. Engineers tend to be zoomed in. Back in my coaching days, these were the clients who kept a detailed journal of their workouts with every rep, set, and weight accounted for and could tell you the exact workout they did on January 4, 2010, along with detailed notes about how they performed that day. Engineers get granular and rely heavily on measurable outsourced information (outsourcing is a key concept I'll talk about in Chapter 8). My Engineer clients wanted clearly stated outcomes, explanations for why they'd be doing things, and details on how both progression and regression would be measured. I gave them spreadsheets with reps, sets, times, and expected progressions from week to week, not because physiology works that way but because it put their minds at ease. Many times, Engineers would stick to the exact plan because that's how I wrote it.

The upside of Engineers is that they tend to make decisions based on evidence and have clear ways to measure progress and regression. If they decide to track their food, they eat right to the calorie. When they commit to a health regimen, they execute it with exactitude for whatever duration of time they do it. The downside is that Engineers can get fixated on small details and miss the big picture. Take, for example, the client who got worried about day-to-day HRV from back in Chapter 6. They got overly worried about the dip in their HRV score without understanding that this sign of stress was an indicator of effective training. The lesson we can take away from Engineers is the importance of having clearly defined goals and indicators that we track with some regularity so that we can identify patterns and don't get caught by surprise.

Intuitives, on the other hand, are feelers. They care less about numbers and data. Intuitives place more value on their internal sense of how things are going. While they may use devices, they're going to make the final decision based on their gut. When I would program for Intuitive athletes, I didn't give them strict day-to-day programs because I learned that if I wasn't standing right there, they did what they wanted anyway. Instead, I programmed a menu of options that were constrained by the goal of that day, week, or cycle but allowed for a lot of freedom to make decisions based on how they were feeling. Intuitives rely on insourcing, information from their own experience (another concept I'll talk about in more detail in Chapter 8). This often allows them a more robust mindset when they don't get the exact outcome they expected.

The upside is that Intuitives don't get stuck zoomed in. They sense the big picture and don't let small details push them around as long as they feel like they're headed in the right direction. The downside is that Intuitives can get stuck zoomed out and become bewildered by their lack of progress or even worsening of the problem they are trying to solve or the goal they're trying to achieve. Intuitives are also more likely to take shortcuts and have a "good enough" attitude. Being an Intuitive doesn't lead to laziness per se (although an Engineer might see it differently), but it can create a laissez-faire attitude when it comes to making things happen. In the context of health and performance longevity, this sometimes sets up Intuitives for failure before they even start because they don't clearly state the desired outcomes, making it impossible for them to know if they are making any progress.

Most people are not firmly planted in one category or the other but fall somewhere toward one end of this spectrum. You might even be more of one type in some circumstances and more of the other in other circumstances. For example, you could be metric driven and strict when it comes to finances but loose and intuitive when it comes to how you take care of your body—or vice versa. The balance between the two shifts dynamically, but the goal is to minimize the swing of the pendulum and keep it toward the middle. Where you fall on the continuum may also color which types of indicators and tools you are naturally drawn to. Engineers may prefer to track heart rate precisely during every cardiovascular training session and count the steps of every walk, whereas Intuitives might use approximations like perceived exertion or a route through the neighborhood plus or minus a detour if something looks interesting.

Being either an Engineer or an Intuitive is not necessarily a predictor of success or failure in regard to performance longevity but instead may provide a heads-up about where failure points might arise. Be aware of which direction you tend to lean so you can be on guard against the downsides and leverage the upsides.

SELF-REFLECTION QUESTIONS

Where do you fall on the continuum of Engineer and Intuitive in general? With your health and performance?

Does the context affect where you sit on the continuum? For example, you're more of an Engineer with money but less as a parent.

Ask some people who are close to you if they agree. Why or why not?

Where are those people on the continuum? How do you know?

SYSTEMS > DISCIPLINE

All of this dashboard and toolkit stuff sounds nice, but how are you supposed to put together feasible units of action in the real world?

If you browse social media or watch YouTube, you may have noticed a trend toward discipline. There is no shortage of characters telling people to tighten up and get disciplined. On one hand, I get it. This is a natural balancing of the scales against the licentious and wayward behavior that accompanies some perceptions of modern Western culture. Instant gratification has not been good for us at large, and personal responsibility must be a core part of the answer. This same philosophy gets misdirected toward failures in health behavior. That is a wholesale misunderstanding of the problem, in my experience. Doing it "because you're supposed to" is the attitude of people who already do it. Discipline, strictly speaking, is obedience to rules, whether those rules were self-imposed or administered by an authority.

The life cycle of discipline requires mental energy to not break the rules, and that energy is, like all energy used by people, finite. When I talk to individuals who seem disciplined, I usually find two things behind the curtain:

- First, the most rigid among them are Engineers. They have proclivities that drive them toward higher degrees of conscientiousness.

- Second, and more important for our broader discussion, they have systems in place. The fittest, healthiest people I know organize their lives so that they are pushed toward habits that create the outcomes they want. When they wake up in the morning, their running shoes are by the door with the socks they're going to wear already stuck inside them. They don't buy a family-sized jar of peanut butter and then stare at it hoping they don't eat the whole thing; they just don't buy peanut butter in the first place.

Brushing your teeth and bathing yourself are tasks that do not require discipline. Your parents likely gave you a system for these tasks when you were a kid, and you probably use that same system now. You can do the same for other areas of performance longevity by adopting a systems approach.

Building good systems for performance longevity is about setting yourself up for success by organizing your environment and your habits to point you in the direction you want to go so you don't have to spend expensive cognitive energy thinking about it. For example, as I write this book on my laptop, my phone is turned off and in another room entirely. I could leave it on in my office and just try to have the discipline not to look at it, but I find it more effective and reliable to have a system in place.

Talking about systems is one thing, but producing them is another, and it doesn't have to be difficult. In fact, the simpler and easier your system is to start, the more likely you are to use the indicators and tools that you've selected. A big reason I ask you to perform personal health experiments in the workbook is that I want you to tinker with a variety of indicators and tools to see if and how they might fit into *your* system. Putting items and reminders in your environment is a good place to begin.

Mise en place ("everything in its place") is a culinary term used to describe the act of getting all of the ingredients out and in one place before you start to cook. I encourage you to adopt this same approach when it comes to your personal health experiments. If, as part of a sleep experiment, you're going to try rolling on a foam roller every night before bed, don't put the thing across the hall or on the other side of the house. Put it right next to your bed so that, as you wind down, there is almost zero friction between you and the behavior you're trying to change.

This preparedness leads to the kind of consistency that gets results. That's true even if a specific tool or indicator you're trying out doesn't end up working for you. If you find that a recipe isn't to your liking, putting the ingredients out before you cook still makes cooking that dish a smoother and more organized process. As a buddy of mine who is former military says, "Right tools. Right place. Right time." This works for teaching young soldiers and sailors to be more organized with their efforts, and it can help you, too.

Building systems to help keep you on track works on the micro level, like putting a foam roller near the bed, but it works on the macro level, too. Coordinating strategies for MIND, MVMT, and MTTR on a larger scale starts to build a lifestyle of performance longevity. Seemingly small but consistent habits will synergize into the net effect of lifelong vitality. In Chapter 8, we'll take everything you've learned so far and amalgamate it into a personal health system that not only keeps the check engine light off but also keeps the engine tuned and humming.

The best system I've found that predicts overall performance longevity is learning through an experimental mindset.

SELF-REFLECTION QUESTIONS

Think about systems you've already built in your life that make it easier to do the things you're supposed to do. These things, when organized well, make life run smoother. It could be which spouse or partner handles the money, how you organize household chores or automotive maintenance, or maybe the way you keep a carry-on packed for frequent work travel.

_____

_____

Were these systems always in place, or did they come from lessons learned?

_____

_____

What time, energy, and/or frustration do they save you now that they're in place?

_____

_____

Maybe some have even helped you achieve a specific goal. If so, how?

_____

_____

What is one simple thing you could do today to start building a system for performance longevity overall?

_____

_____

Think of some tools and indicators that you use for your health. How could you organize your use of those things to make it smoother and more efficient?

_____

_____

Here's an easy example from my friend coach Paul Sharp. Paul gets up at an ungodly hour of the morning to get his cardio in before work. To keep on track with his nutrition, he sets out his supplements and his first meal before he goes to bed. Rather than rely on willpower alone, he puts things in their place so they're ready when he needs them.

CHAPTER 8: | Developing a Personal Health System

> **"** *The ideal is unnatural naturalness, or natural unnaturalness. I mean it is a combination of both. I mean here is natural instinct and here is control. You are to combine the two in harmony. Not if you have one to the extreme, you'll be very unscientific. If you have another to the extreme, you become, all of a sudden, a mechanical man—no longer a human being. It is a successful combination of both. That way it is a process of continuing growth.*"
>
> **—Bruce Lee**

All this talk about building systems, KPIs, dashboards, and toolkits can make performance longevity sound like an impossibly complicated engineering problem, but it doesn't have to be. In fact, the most sustainable practices like those we discussed in Section Two and explore more deeply in the workbook, are often simple and direct. More than having a scattering of isolated habits, indicators, and tools, it can be a cohesive approach to sustaining the behavior that supports health.

I think that's an important distinction that requires a bit more clarification. Health is not a static state of being free of disease that is maintained by luck, genetics, and modern medicine. The maintenance and repair of your life vehicle involves knowledge and skills that you learn through practice. They are embodied. The longer and more intentionally you practice the necessary skills, the easier it gets to refine both your dashboard and your toolkit. The maintenance of health or, more specifically, performance longevity pays dividends to everything you care about in life.

You may have noticed that I haven't outlined any specific protocols in this book. While prescribed lists of "do this, then do that" can be helpful as starting points or illustrations of effect, they won't help you engage in the most robust and reliable health behavior of all-continuous learning. I don't mean learning in the sense of collecting various menu items to choose from to maintain your body and mind, though that can be part of it. Learning in the deepest sense is not merely the collection of data; it's the development of a robust set of skills that lead you closer to being self-determined in the way you approach your health. My primary goal and greatest joy as a coach is to make an autonomous athlete. Being an autonomous caretaker of your performance longevity doesn't mean you're on your own and there's no help. It means you can take what you've learned, spin it around in the centrifuge of your mind, pull out the parts that are most meaningful to you, and then use them to draw your own informed conclusions. No matter how good health technology gets, nothing can be healthy *for* you. You have to do it yourself.

This final chapter synthesizes the ideas we've explored into a cohesive philosophy, leading directly into the real learning: the workbook. This is where you will really start to apply the concepts discussed throughout this text. In fact, you could probably stop here and flip to the workbook if you wanted to. What follows in this chapter will certainly help tie a nice bow on the concepts, lead you into the X's and O's of how to perform the experiments, and hopefully save you some heartache. But could you just start doing the experiments that are in the workbook and improve your health and performance? Heck yeah, you could. In fact, when I work with clients, I don't give them a long philosophical dissertation before we get to work. We just get started, and over time the concepts naturally begin to sink in as a consequence of the work we are doing.

SELF-REFLECTION QUESTIONS

Write down an example of a long-term change you have made that has had a positive impact on your health and/or performance. This could be in regard to something at work or at home.

_____

_____

How did you know that an adjustment was necessary? What metrics got your attention?

_____

_____

Why did the change that you made work for you? Be specific.

_____

_____

What adjustments did you have to make to fit this change into your life?

_____

_____

What are some other things you've tried that were less successful?

_____

_____

Why weren't they successful?

_____

_____

What metrics were in place that let you know the impact of this change? Were there any blind spots in your approach that limited your results?

_____

_____

SUSTAINABLE CHANGE

Over the course of my career, I've always had a bias toward sustainability. Being good for a day doesn't mean a whole lot from my point of view. While there is some merit to the saying "you only have to win the gold one time," behind that one time is a history of doing the right things that culminate in that moment. Furthermore, the most revered among us are the ones who not only get on top but stay on top. Why? Because it is difficult to stay consistent over time. We get complacent, we forget things, life and responsibilities get in the way. For these reasons, long-term behavior, especially long-term health behavior, is one of the hardest things for many of us to change for the positive.

I've had the opportunity to work on some health technology applications, and outside of basic functionality, one of the biggest questions for developers is how to get people to keep using the technology. Even when the technology is helping them. Most of the time, the answers to the question of how to keep people engaged with their health include things like gamification, education in the form of daily factoids and trivia, continual upgrades for novelty, and reduced user interface friction. While these things certainly have their place, they don't quite cut it when it comes to creating sustainable changes in health. Gamifying health can be helpful to some degree. Rules of play, scores, and competition all motivate people to engage with the intended environment, whether it be as part of an employee incentive program or a health technology. Novelty can help, too. We see this a lot with the internet and especially social media platforms but sometimes as part of fitness facilities as well: new equipment, exercises, classes, and programs. TikTok videos promote new exercises or new takes on old exercises. You'd think that in a culture of neophiles, the newness would keep us on board. But again, it doesn't. Some approaches even aim to inform. Podcasts, books (ironically), and to some degree the ol' television provide free and direct information about all of the latest and greatest in research and practice in health and performance. The quality of that information aside, we are the most informed culture in history, but also the least healthy. Maybe information alone isn't the answer.

In my experience, if you want to have the best shot at long-term change and, even better, you want ownership of the process of change, nothing is better than education. *Wait, Rob, didn't you just say that information isn't the answer?* Yes. But the delivery of information is not the same thing as education. Education comes from the Latin *educaré,* which means to bring out. A real education brings forth understanding from inside a person. From inside *you.* A true education about your personal longevity cannot be delivered by any podcast, app, website, seminar, or online class; it comes from the purposeful cultivation of your own experience. Through meaningful engagement in your own process. Legitimate aids in this outcome facilitate, guide, and direct you in the process of cultivating your own path up the mountain. As my friend and super coach Kenny Kane says, "Really good coaches and teachers are sherpas."

Historically, I'm not a video game person. We had the original Nintendo in my house when I was a little kid, and once in a while I'd give it a whirl, but it was never my thing. My entire life I've been more of a gym rat and a go-outside kinda guy. This winter, though, there was a hiccup in that track record when my daughter gave my wife and me a Nintendo Switch along with the game *The Legend of Zelda: Breath of the Wild* for Christmas. First released in 2017, *Breath of the Wild* is one of the best-selling and widely considered one the best games ever made. I have to admit, it got me. I had never played a game through to the end, but I played this game nearly every night for two and a half months until I reached the crescendo and defeated the final boss.

As a person who as a rule has zero interest in video games, I was curious about what made me stick to this one. Was it the graphics? The gamification? Were they tickling my damnable dopamine censors against my better judgment? What made this game so popular? One of the major attractors for me, that has been widely corroborated through research on Nintendo message boards, is that *Breath of the Wild* is an open-world game. Within the technological constraints of the system and the geographical constraints of the world, the world is mostly free to explore in whatever way the player chooses. You can climb mountains, go hunting, catch wild horses, swim in rivers, pursue a variety of side quests, discover tools, and interact with other characters in a myriad of ways. You can work through the game in somewhat of an order, or you can bounce around as you see fit. *Breath of the Wild* offers multiple ways to surmount challenges and solve puzzles in the game. There are no instructions, no step-by-steps, and no right or wrong ways to do it. You simply play and explore.

This flexibility is what keeps people coming back to this game. A quick search on Reddit or YouTube will plunge you into a community that loves this game and its mythology. They play it again and again in different modes and even add their own rules and constraints to see what happens. By the end of 2023, *Breath of the Wild* had sold 33.3 million copies. If it was a music album, it would be the second best-selling album of all time, just behind Michael Jackson's *Thriller.*

This anecdote reveals a deeper lesson than how to get people excited about a video game. It demonstrates that autonomy is a deep motivator of human behavior. Choosing your own adventure is an intrinsic part of what makes you human. When you feel a sense of control over the direction of your life, you develop confidence and a sense of progress and growth. These qualities provide you with robust tools, concepts, and frameworks that you develop yourself. The road to autonomy and self-determination is not through the delivery of rote protocols and action items, but through a continuous self-directed process of exploration.

What exactly does all of that have to do with performance longevity? Am I saying that podcasts and protocols are a waste of time and that the solution is a Zelda-quality video game that can keep you properly hooked so you'll always pay attention to your dashboard? No. What I am saying is that you need opportunities to practice, experiment, and adjust.

T(H)INKERERS

The people I know who have performed at a high level over the course of years and even decades are tinkerers and thinkers. They are always trying things, tweaking things, challenging themselves, and reforming their health and performance practices. Tinkering means "I'm gonna try this to see what happens and be open to the possibilities." These high achievers also think and reflect on the things they've tried over time in order to improve their understanding of what's going in their minds and bodies. One of the hidden benefits of constantly tinkering to improve your performance longevity is that it keeps your health and performance tab open on the web browser of your mind.

You might remember my "car buddy" from the introduction to this book. He was always changing out the tires, tweaking the engine, or putting on a new exhaust, or refurbishing the interior of his truck. If I had a question about which tires to put on my truck, he knew what to recommend because he'd tried most of them. It was the same for shocks, brake pads, and just about anything related to the function of an automobile. He knew every inch of his vehicles, what all of the noises were, what things might give us issues if we drove on the beach, and what tools to bring along just in case. He knew how his truck would handle in the mountains versus on the sand and how to adjust for the road conditions. Not coincidentally, his vehicles always ran well, not necessarily because he did any one thing in particular or all at once but because he was always "in it." His mind was attuned to his vehicles. Their care and maintenance was continuously a part of his thinking as a course of habit.

This same attitude toward tinkering for health can carry you a long way. It doesn't mean a lack of commitment to a set of metrics, bouncing around from one thing to another. As already discussed, too cavalier an approach can fail to yield measurable results that you can actually learn from. Instead, tinkering provides an introduction to the attitude of trying things out. It is the most rudimentary form of science. Some people call it *play.* Learning to play with the different nuts and bolts that move the needle of your health turns it into a bit of a game that you can stay engaged with for the long haul, which is the entire goal of pursuing performance longevity.

SELF-REFLECTION QUESTIONS

Write down an example of a long-term change you have made that has had a positive impact on your health and/or performance. This could be in regard to something at work or at home.

How did you know that an adjustment was necessary? What metrics got your attention?

Why did it work for you? Be specific.

What adjustments did you have to make to fit this change into your life?

What are some other things you've tried that were less successful?

_____

_____

Why weren't they successful?

_____

_____

What metrics were in place that let you know the results? Were there any blind spots in your approach that limited your results?

_____

_____

Think of a protocol for health or performance that sounds good but that you can't figure out exactly how to make fit into your life. What would you have to change to make it work? Be specific.

_____

_____

What could you alter about that protocol to try it without making any lifestyle changes?

_____

_____

Think of a meaningful learning experience you've had (in any realm, not just performance longevity) that led you to a deeper level of understanding and resulted in a measurable change in you.

_____

_____

What made that particular experience meaningful? What made this moment click?

_____

_____

Many times these sorts of experiences seem to find you randomly. What steps could you take to make any learning you decide to undertake more meaningful to you?

_____

_____

When a MVMT indicator flashes on your dashboard, what tool do you use to address it?

_____

_____

Where does that tool fit in the R3 model and the proximal-to-distal model?

_____

_____

Is there a better tool you could be using?

_____

_____

If you don't know, what reliable resource could you consult to find out about the tools that are available?

_____

_____

TUNING THE HUMAN

It would be nearly impossible to count how many times over the course of my career I have been asked questions like these:

- "Which stretches are the best ones for me to do?"
- "What breathing technique should I use?"
- "What's the best way to put on muscle?"

To which my answer would often be, "Let's find out together." While I'm happy to provide starting points, thinking that that starting point will sustain your changing needs over time is a mistake. Over reliance on protocols often makes for a fragile approach that ultimately leads to frustration and failure when it comes to the deployment of tools. That is because if the "answer" is delivered to you, there is no learning involved. If some sense of personal ownership and understanding doesn't underpin the why, when, and how of the indicators and tools you choose, they won't last. You don't need to become a subject matter expert in psychology, exercise, or biochemistry to glean the benefits of these things, either. But you do have to become an expert in *what works for you* if you want the habits of performance longevity to stick.

Developing an experimental mindset is about having the willingness to try things out and see what happens. It may be easier to offload some of the cognitive burden to rote protocols in the short term, but over the long haul, an experimental mindset is far more robust because you become a conscious participant in your own adaptive process. When you take on the mantra "Let's see what happens," you find solutions that work for you in the context of your own life. That's not to say there aren't any objective realities or that you shouldn't use metrics. I hope I've done a good enough job throughout this book making the opposing case. By experimenting with solutions within the confines of established science, you can find out how to apply performance longevity solutions that are meaningful to you.

When the solutions to your health and performance problems make sense and fit within the framework of your perception and the context of your life, you buy in more completely and sustain focus on them long enough for deeper and more lasting changes to occur. Interestingly, this has become a hot topic of discussion in computer science labs in the last handful of years. Health apps are a large business sector estimated at between $60 and $80 billion in 2023 and are expected to grow by leaps and bounds in the coming years. One of the hardest things to accomplish in human-computer interaction (HCI), especially in regard to health is, as I mentioned earlier in this chapter, getting people to keep engaging in health behavior.

The research of m. c. schraefel and associates of the University of Southampton in the UK has greatly influenced my thinking in this regard. What schraefel found in researching health technology adherence is deeply informative about the topics I am discussing in this chapter. In a paper entitled "Experiment in a Box (XB): An Interactive Technology Framework for Sustainable Health Practices," published in *Frontiers in Computer Science,* schraefel and her colleagues show that an experimental framework "supports user autonomy and competence" and that "participants develop health practices from the interventions that are still in use long after the intervention is finished." That means an experimental approach to health and performance yielded better long-term results than the insertion of a standard protocol.

Why? schraefel found that more participants took ownership over their own processes and developed "knowledge, skill, and practices" that made them feel capable of interpreting information regarding the exploration of their own health. When we go through a process of exploration, we find more meaning in the things we learn. This is true for all of life, so why would performance longevity be any different? This experimental mindset does not have to occur without outside help. Looking to subject matter experts and resources in healthcare, fitness, and performance is often necessary to find reliable starting places. But no advice or prescription is a substitute for your own experience. schraefel calls this the "insourcing-outsourcing continuum."

You may remember that in Chapter 7, I introduced these terms when describing Engineers and Intuitives. Engineers like to outsource data: *What are the clear-cut measurables?* Intuitives tend to insource information: *How does what I'm feeling reflect what's going on?* The process of sliding between the two is an art that is honed over time, and if you learn to calibrate your perception through the skill of insourcing and outsourcing, you can become more greatly attuned to what the signals from your body and mind are truly communicating to you. And in doing so, you can become a finely tuned machine of performance longevity.

In a final tip of the hat to m. c. schraefel and her coauthor, Dr. Eric Hekler of UC San Diego, I'll talk about a term they coined that beautifully sums up this entire sentiment and provides a North Star for us moving forward. They use the word "tuning" (from a paper of the same name) to describe the process of continual adjustment, akin to tuning a musical instrument or engine. Tuning is the "ability to select and adapt appropriate KSP {knowledge, skills, and practices} to build and maintain health and well-being across contexts." Being well tuned means that all of the parts are working together to create synergy in their outcomes. This is true for instruments, machines, and human beings. You are in a constant state of adapting to the pressures of your environments (including your choices). Mostly, these adaptive processes happen without any conscious participation on your part. Tuning is a constant state of awareness and adjustment—in other words, tweaking, tinkering, and experimenting to see what makes you "sound better."

Learning to tune in to your health and performance is not a one-time deal any more than it is with a musical instrument. If you want to play your best, you have to tune the instrument over and over again. It's a constant cycle of listening, adjusting, and playing. Being in tune is also relative to the environment. If you play in a band, it's about the harmony of all of the players, not just one person. The process of tuning an instrument, machine, or human is also a constant fight against detuning. That is simply the order of nature. Even when things seem static, subtle effects are taking place that are attempting to pull your system out of tune. Knowing that things fall apart is the rule of the road keeps you vigilant so you can stay a step ahead and keep performing your best. To keep your instrument in tune, *you* must tune it.

Tuning in to your internal frequency of health is continuous and is even affected by what song and genre you want to play. Maybe you have a short-term goal of running a 5K or a marathon. Or perhaps you're stressed because your in-laws are staying in your extra bedroom for two weeks. You might even have a vacation planned where you know your eating habits may take a hit. Any of these may require some fine-tuning to maintain health and performance in the new context presented. If you're going to have to get up early before work to get your run training in, you may have to give additional attention to getting to bed on time with monastic consistency. In-laws in town may mean more rigorous scheduling to offset interruptions to daily household rhythms or planning specific times to organize your thoughts. If your eating habits are going to be disrupted during travel, planning self-regulation strategies ahead of time can be very helpful (eating dessert no more than twice that week or putting constraints on alcohol). Ultimately, the point is to stay flexible in your approach so you can adjust your habits, practices, and methods however you might need to. There's no singular, absolute state of perfection whether you're in total control of your routine or some external challenge or unforeseen circumstance arises. The process is, as I've said in many ways in this chapter, the development of a skill that occurs with intentional practice.

While the process of tuning offers a wonderful 10,000-foot view of how you can orient your intentions for the long-term maintenance of your health, an important question remains:

How do you actually do it?

Improving your ability to tune your mind and body is not brought about by reading, or watching videos, or talking about it; it comes from trying things for yourself and learning from them. In other words, through thoughtful experimentation.

PERSONAL HEALTH EXPERIMENTS

Everything I've talked about up to now has led to this very important point. The concepts explored in this book are helpful for understanding how to manage health and performance over the long haul, but what matters most is using them. The personal health experiments found in the workbook (and hopefully the ones you later create for yourself) offer you a way to do just that. There are examples in the workbook from each of the M3 Model categories (MIND, MoVeMenT, and MaTTeR) to help you get started, but this is a process that can and should continue forever. If you engage in these experiments, you'll have some foundational habits for building your dashboard of indicators and your toolbox. These personal health experiments can serve as a springboard for a more organized approach to building a robust and sustainable personal health practice for a lifetime.

Let me set the stage for these experiments. A good place to start is what they are not. Personal health experiments are not blind human randomized control trials performed under laboratory conditions. It is wholly impossible to create laboratory conditions in real life. Laboratory conditions involved high degrees of control over research subjects and the interventions used. Measurement tools are rigorously calibrated, and outcome measures undergo statical analysis to determine whether the findings are valid. This just is not possible for everyday life. There are two key things to take away from this, however:

Don't take your experience (or anybody else's) as gospel. In fact, a good habit is to look for ways in which your initial impression might be wrong or incomplete. Attempting to take apart your own hypotheses is a helpful habit even if you're not a research scientist. It keeps you honest and more aware of your biases. This is also where the insourcing-outsourcing continuum helps.

Additionally, in good research the investigators not only may find outcomes that inform future practice, but also use what they found to propose directions for further investigation. You should do the same. This pursuit of curiosity about how to effectively improve your own well-being will pay off in spades over the long haul.

Now let's talk about what these experiments are. The interventions you'll use are supported by science and experience. They also are opportunities to develop heuristics that let you know which indicators and tools best work for you so that you can make quick, increasingly accurate decisions about how you manage your health and performance. The personal health experiments in the workbook also offer opportunities for self-reflection, a core component of long-term health behavior. Not just what works, but what works *for you.*

Use the experiments provided in the workbook as a jumping-off point, and return to them from time to time to see if anything has changed. Things that don't produce a result for you now may be effective next month or next year. More important than these specific experiments is that you continue to try things on your own and develop new insights and hypotheses that support and test your performance longevity. Over time, this builds the habits you'll need to become a more calibrated tuner of your own body and mind.

Personal Health Experiment Story

Tom is fifty-seven years old. He's gotten between seven and seven and a half hours of sleep every night but wakes up feeling groggy and stiff. Tom is so groggy in the morning, in fact, that his wife knows not to ask him any questions until after his third cup of coffee, unless of course she wants to ask the same question a couple of hours later.

Tom is an avid college basketball fan, and one Sunday while scrolling through the ESPN app, he came across an article about sleep extension research for college basketball players. A Stanford researcher had done a seven-year study examining the effects of extended sleep in performance metrics for basketball. The data that was compiled showed clearly that players who slept longer jumped higher, shot more accurately, and ran faster. In addition, they even reported improvements in mood (something Tom's wife would really appreciate).

Tom thought that if it was good enough for Stanford basketball, it was good enough for him to try. Besides, he could use the new Apple Watch he'd gotten the previous Christmas to monitor his sleep and keep him on track. He wasn't sure he could get to sleep two hours earlier, so he decided to give an hour extra a try for at least a week.

Every night for the next week, Tom went to bed half an hour earlier and woke up half an hour later. At first he wasn't sure it was going to make much of a difference, but after a couple days, he noticed something— he was drinking less coffee. He was more alert when he woke up, and the low-back stiffness that he'd thought was just a normal part of being in his fifties was greatly reduced and almost gone by the time he was done walking his dogs.

Did Tom experience the same level of change in performance as those young basketball stars? No. But now Tom was curious about what else he could improve if he tried.

RESEARCH YOUR OWN EXPERIENCE

At the beginning of this journey, I used the imagery of driving along and suddenly having your car conk out with the engine smoking, stranding you on the side of the road. In this scenario, you had ignored the indicator lights. For one reason or another, you passed over the signs and signals that might have kept you out of trouble, and all of the back interest on those decisions came due at once. It's obvious that this isn't a good idea with cars or with money, so, to avoid those kinds of situations, we lean on habits and technology that often get shared with us. Sometimes that is necessary, but not at the behest of our own informed judgment.

Far too few of us are equipped to care for the bodies and minds that we must use to navigate life. The goal of this book is to equip you with a skill set to make you more capable in the care of your mind and body so that you can do your best at whatever it is you care about most. I've used the concepts outlined here to help everyone from Navy SEALs and world champions to regular folks like you and me to stay on the long road of performance longevity. If you apply them consistently, they can work for you, too.

The first step is organizing the way you pay attention. Do you know what your signals (KPIs) are? Do you know the information your signals are conveying? Are they telling you about something that is coming (leading indicators) or something that has already happened (lagging indicators)? As you pay more attention, you're building a Performance Longevity Dashboard. Like any dashboard, your Performance Longevity Dashboard gives you important information so that you can stay aware of what's going on and make good decisions. In this case, it's not so much about constant tracking and hypervigilance over every health marker, but instead about the net effect of how your body and mind are functioning as a whole.

The indicators for the dashboard can be organized into the three buckets of MIND, MoVeMenT, and MaTTeR. Within each of these categories are a nearly infinite number of indicators. In Section Two, I presented some examples for each category that are founded on legitimate research as well as the best practices I've seen and used over my career. Please do not take these examples as gospel but instead as places to start experimenting.

Information alone is not enough; after gathering that information, you must have a course of action. Knowing your car needs work doesn't help much if you don't have the tools to do something about it. Building a toolkit that helps you prevent and resolve issues is just as essential as knowing what's going on. But selecting tools can be tricky because the marketplace of health and wellness often relies on the consumer's lack of expertise to sell tools that purport to but often do not actually deliver performance longevity.

Having clear guidelines that help you decide which tools to include in your Performance Longevity Toolkit can save you time and energy. Back in Chapter 3, I talked about my buddy Mickey Schuch and how his R3 Model of robust, reliable, and repeatable systems can be applied to the way you think about the kinds of tools you want to bring into your health toolkit:

- Robust tools are hard to break and will stand up to the demands of your lifestyle.

- Reliable tools will deliver as promised.

- Repeatability means that the operation and deployment of the tool are clear enough to you that you can use it properly to get the results you want over and over again.

Within this R3 Model, you also want to select tools from proximal to distal. Which tools will you keep close to you, and which ones will you keep on the periphery? Tools being proximal or distal has nothing to do with their efficacy but rather relates to your access to and understanding of them. Proximal tools are what you have close by and therefore are the ones you should spend more time and energy understanding because you will rely on them the most.

Collecting and collating indicators and tools to maintain performance longevity doesn't have to be a complicated or arduous process. There's no rush. Begin with one thing from one of the M3 categories that you're sure you can track and change and go for it. Then tinker around and see what happens. If you're more of an Engineer, you may be attracted to easily quantifiable data, such as daily monitoring of your resting heart rate and heart rate variability. If you're an Intuitive, you might pick indicators that are based on an internal sense of change, such as the quality of your breathing when you perform Sun Salutation. One type isn't better than the other. There's a constant interplay between information you get from outside of you (outsourcing) and information you corroborate internally (insourcing). To move reliably toward performance longevity, you need both. The indicators you use should have standards of comparison that make them valid and reliable. With that said, don't mistake the forest for the trees. Remember—zoom in for clarity, zoom out for understanding.

With time and practice, you'll find anchor points around which you can experiment. Sleep may be a critical metric you are in tune with on a constant basis, but you might tinker with different tools that affect how and when you sleep. That could mean trying a sleep supplement or stretching before bed. As you experiment more and more, you'll engage in the process of tuning, where you make small tweaks and adjustments on a regular basis to keep things humming. This ability to stay in tune with the context of life demands molds you into a conscious participant in the process of your adaptation—which, just like the wear-and-tear of an engine, will happen whether you pay attention to it or not. At least with the former, there are fewer unwanted surprises, and when challenges do show up, you'll have a better chance of sustaining your performance through those challenges.

My sincere hope for you after you engage with the material in this book is that it will become an integrated philosophy for how you think about maintaining your health—that these concepts and ideas become so second nature to you that you nearly forget what they are called unless someone wanting to know how you stay so darn consistent with your health practices asks you about them. Don't become too anchored on any one example that we have explored. Ask yourself, *What's under the surface here?* If there's a specific indicator or tool that works well for you and continues to do so over time, fantastic. But I do hope you'll keep, as Bruce Lee said, "researching your own experience."

 ## AUTONOMY AND OWNERSHIP

Client G was referred to me because, like many of my new clients, he was desperate. G was a young active-duty sailor who, let's just say, is a doer of very dangerous things. He had suffered a debilitating back injury followed by an experimental surgery. The prognosis was that he'd be forced to be medically discharged from the military in the prime of his life—a nocebic blow to his state of mind, no doubt.

When we started working together, even the simplest tasks were a shot in the dark for G. His walking was effortful. He struggled to get up and down off the ground. He could not stabilize his spine purposefully, nor could the segments of his spine tolerate variability. He received poor scores on key markers for general health, never mind elite military service.

We began with some basic rehabilitative movements to reduce his pain and gradually improve his ability to tolerate motion. Over time, G progressed (as measured by MVMT indicators, of course) to more and more emphasis on performance development for tasks specific to his operational duties. As I write this, a man who at one time could not get out of his truck without pain can work while wearing his full military kit.

For all intents and purposes, G's tenacity and discipline combined with a decent plan saved his career. Although this tale demonstrates the incredible healing power of the human body if given the proper opportunities, that's not the moral of this particular story. The moral here is that not only is this young man now able to perform his job, but he better understands his own needs.

More recently, G has taken over the majority of his own fitness training and care. On a check-in call, we discussed what he was up to. What I found remarkable, other than the horrible inaccuracy of the original prognosis, was how many of the more rudimentary exercises G had curated as formal movement indicators for his daily readiness. Furthermore, he had married those to exercises, stretches, and therapies that he figured out would keep him ahead of the game. He now has the tools he needs to effectively tune his own physiology.

PERFORMANCE LONGEVITY AS A LIFESTYLE

As you get better and better at purposefully building systems that support your performance longevity and keep you in tune, you'll find that more and more, they'll overlap and support each other. Before you know it, tuning in to your indicators and deploying tools to test out personal health hypotheses will be a matter of constant practice. When this happens, you create a running audit that gives you a stream of information about what's going on with mind and body. You'll be sensitive to acute changes in feel and function. Furthermore, when issues pop up, whether small or large, you will be able to more successfully alter your strategies to stay on track. You'll be more attuned to things like whether you need more or better-quality sleep, how you're responding to your stress load, and the most appropriate use of available tools in the circumstance. If you've built your systems on sound indicators, your sensitivities will be informed by real metrics that inform and challenge your biases.

When performance longevity becomes a lifestyle, you don't just think about the first-order effects of your health and performance choices. You will no longer think only about the immediate effects things like stress, exercise, and sleep. You will more carefully consider how the signals and the way you respond to them reflect your health and performance trajectory into the future. Developing knowledge and skills in performance longevity is not a final destination but an invitation to learn and explore—to take the information you get, whether it's from a wearable, a movement practice, an article, or a healthcare provider, and filter it through your own informed understanding of your personal explorations. This kind of philosophy offers you the most powerful outcome you can achieve: autonomy over your own health and performance.

The skills and practices offered in this book are meant as a scaffolding for you to build upon. I hope that the concepts, ideas, and experiments I've proposed will provide you with a sound structure for the development of your own sustainable personal health system. Applied thoughtfully, these concepts are foundational to the long-term pursuit of health, performance, and vitality. I've seen them work for the highest-performing humans among us and some of the most wounded, too. I'm certain that if you give them an earnest try, they'll lead you toward a better understanding of your needs and the ability to more competently pursue your own health solutions.

Thanks for reading,

Rob Wilson

> **“** *Any fool can know. The point is to understand.* ”
>
> —**Albert Einstein**

THE CHECK ENGINE LIGHT WORKBOOK

Welcome to the Check Engine Light Workbook. This workbook is designed to directly support the learning of the concepts outlined in the main part of the book.

You may have noticed that while Section Two, which covers the M3 Model, shares some examples of indicators and tools, there are no outright recommendations. I'll briefly explain why, as it is relevant to what you really care about: being healthier and performing better over the long haul.

As I said in Chapter 8, performance longevity is not something that can be given to you as a supplement, protocol, or medicine. Those sorts of things are helpful for solving some short-term problems, but they are not what sustains a robust existence.

In this twenty-first century, information is more abundant than ever. We are inundated with news stories, social media posts, YouTube videos, podcasts, books, magazines, and newsletters that all vie for our attention, each spouting its claims with equal vigor regardless of the validity or nuance of those claims. It's an attention marketplace. So where does that leave you and what you want? Often, it leaves you stranded. The most difficult part of dealing with the information age is navigating through the fog toward a path that leads you where it is that *you* want to go. That's why the goal of the book and specifically this workbook is to help you learn to think critically about your own performance longevity and which indicators and tools will work best *for you*.

I'll provide some starting points here, but ultimately it will be up to you to expand on the ideas and experience you gain from the work you do with this material. I hope it can continue to serve as a sort of home base whenever you get a bit lost.

The concepts on which this workbook is based are grounded in the principles of andragogy and heutagogy—approaches that recognize adults learn best through self-directed exploration and real-world application. That is to say, rather than deliver stale protocols or techniques, I'm offering a path of exploration so that you can learn what works for you and, even more importantly, how to keep figuring out what works for you. With that in mind, allow me to provide some insight on how to use this workbook.

The Personal Health Experiments are the meat and potatoes (or tofu and kale for you plant-based kids) of this entire learning process. You'll find a menu of experiments to choose from, centered around the categories of MIND, MVMT, and MTTR. Each experiment comes with explicit instructions for how to carry it out. As a reminder, I use the term "experiment" loosely here. These are not human randomized control trials run in a laboratory; they are experiential learning opportunities for you to calibrate your perception more effectively.

Also, while the experiments are categorized according to the M3 Model for easy reference, be on the lookout for how focus on one area may affect other areas in ways you may not expect.

The process of building your dashboard and your toolkit does not end when you're done with this workbook. As long as you are operating the body and mind that you have, they will require ongoing tuning. Which means that developing a better awareness of your indicators and maintaining your toolkit is a lifelong process. You can of course continue to cycle through the Personal Health Experiments that I've provided for the rest of your life, but I encourage you to try new things on your own, too.

Before we jump into the experiments, here are a few hints to help you get started:

- Start with an experiment that really interests you. If you're truly curious, you'll be more likely to stick to the plan.

- Invite other people to join in. Changing habits for the better can be tough. Friends, family, and coworkers can offer encouragement and accountability.

- Choose a doable experiment. While I have done my best to make all of the experiments accessible, some just won't match your lifestyle. Find something you can execute.

- Pick something you need. Be honest with yourself about areas that might need improvement and choose an experiment that can help.

As a brief reminder, the most important aspect of these experiments is not how you perform against any single metric. This isn't a test for you to get scored on, nor is it an experiment in a laboratory with rigid controls. These Personal Health Experiments are starting places for you to learn how to pay closer attention to your body, apply some form of key performance indicator to what it is you are feeling or experiencing, and then chart a course forward based on what you've learned about yourself. Use them to build experience fine-tuning your body and mind.

The experiments that follow are listed under each of the categories of the M3 Model: MIND, MVMT, and MTTR. You have three experiments to choose from in each category based on topics discussed in the corresponding chapters in the book. Each of the experiments has a description, which includes the recommended amount of time to devote to it. Additionally, there are both indicators and tools listed for each experiment. Read carefully how to apply those so you have a good experience with the experiment.

There is something here for both the Engineer and the Intuitive. There are indicators that are more granular and measurable, such as heart rate variability, as well as short surveys. Both are important for calibrating perception. Don't underestimate the power of self-reflection that comes from the surveys. They are designed based on conversations I've had with clients, athletes, and students over the last two decades. It was often in these debriefings, as well as in the reflection time afterward, that new understanding about health and performance came to light.

As you engage in these Personal Health Experiments, take care to reflect on the "why" of the measurements and trends you experience. Think carefully, and discuss things with your peers and trusted experts if they're available. The point here is to fully engage in the experiment for the purpose of learning, not simply to complete it in the given time.

GENERAL EXPERIMENT INSTRUCTIONS

Each experiment runs between fifteen and thirty days. Check the bullets at the beginning of each experiment for the minimum run time.

I have provided run times for two reasons. First, they allow enough time for the tools you use to take effect. Second, life happens, and you might need some wiggle room to get the train all the way onto the tracks.

Description

This provides a snapshot of what to expect for the experiment. Be sure to read the full description of the experiment you are doing, as there are nuances to each application.

Each experiment begins with a list that looks like this:

Run time: Number of days the experiment will take; in some cases it is a range

Using experiment indicators: Names of indicators (e.g., HRV, restfulness, surveys), time of day to be recorded, consistency reminder

Using experiment tools: Names of tools and when to use them (e.g., controlled breathing, Sun Salutation, regular bedtime)

Indicators

Each experiment has a set of recommended indicators. Some are qualitative (reflection questions and surveys), and some are quantitative (resting heart rate).

Reflection questions and surveys are provided for each experiment. You will find a starting survey to assess your starting place, a daily survey that helps you reflect and monitor progress along the way, and an ending survey and reflection questions to consider what you've learned.

It's important to use both types of indicators where prompted to. Neither type is more important than the other. Both are essential in calibrating perception and developing awareness.

I went to great effort to make sure that none of the experiments would cause undue time strain, but some of them may require a little forethought for the first few days.

Be consistent with when you measure indicators (for example, in the morning before intervention, post-exercise, etc.). These aren't strict science experiments, but try to standardize the time you record your data each day. For example, when I take my blood pressure for my own health experiments, I do it when I wake up, right after I let my dogs outside to use the bathroom.

This same suggestion applies to your surveys! They're data, too!

Tools

Each experiment also offers some tools to use as interventions of sorts that are directly related to tools I wrote about in the corresponding chapters of the book. For most of the experiments, you may use one tool for the entire period or try different tools, as long as you use each tool for at least five consecutive days. If switching tools, allow a two- to three-day "washout" period before starting the next one.

MIND EXPERIMENTS

Experiment #1: Autonomic Regulation

This experiment is all about learning to tune into your autonomic nervous system (ANS). As discussed in Chapter 3, the ANS is like the accountant for all of the stress that happens in body and mind. Tuning the ANS can have powerful impacts on performance longevity.

In this experiment, you'll have a few different key performance indicators to measure the ANS along with two options for tools to modify it. In addition to the biometric KPIs that are listed, you'll use a stress scale to check in with your perception of stress.

Remember, your overall goal is to calibrate your perception through the use of valid, reliable, and accessible indicators. As you continue to experiment, you'll find the right indicators to put on your dashboard as well as the right tools for your toolkit.

Caution: If you're managing a medical condition, please seek the advice of a trusted healthcare practitioner before you start.

Description

Run time: Fifteen days.

Using experiment indicators: The indicators for this experiment are HRV, blood pressure, resting pulse rate, and a daily stress scale. Choose one of these as your primary indicator and measure it daily at the same time of day. You may use more than one indicator if you want, but maintain a single primary indicator for the entirety of the experiment. For consistency, take measurements first thing in the morning before consuming caffeine or other stimulants and before using the tool.

Using experiment tools: The tools for this experiment are controlled breathing and progressive relaxation. Perform the intervention of your choice at a consistent time of day, adjusting as needed, and stick with it for at least five days.

Indicators

The indicators listed here are arranged from least to most accessible based on cost. If you don't have access to the fanciest one, don't sweat it. Consistency is what matters most.

- **Heart rate variability:** Record this number from your wearable device (if available).

- **Blood pressure:** Monitors are available for $20 to $160. Make sure to write down both the upper (systolic) and the lower (diastolic) numbers.

- **Resting pulse rate:** Move your fingers around on either your wrist or your neck until you feel the *boomp boomp*. That's your pulse. When the clock strikes zero, start counting. Count the total beats in sixty seconds, then record this number.

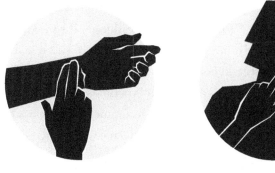

Radial Pulse   Carotid Pulse

- **Daily stress scale:** To be completed in the evening between dinner and bedtime.

- **Bonus:** Perceived stress scale: This questionnaire is a bit longer and can be filled out at the beginning and end of the experiment. Find it in the Resources section of the book.

Tools

Use each tool daily for at least five consecutive days, maintaining a consistent time and setting. To avoid confounding results, use only one tool at a time before switching.

Controlled Breathing

Controlled breathing has a known effect on the autonomic nervous system and stress. Different strategies work for different people, but the following two breathing sequences are generally safe and reliable ways to start exploring. Each sequence represents six breaths per minute. Whichever one you choose, perform the controlled breathing for five to fifteen minutes a day.

- 3:2:5 means to inhale for three seconds, hold for two seconds, and then exhale for five seconds.

- 4:6 means to inhale for four seconds and exhale for six seconds, with no holding other than naturally occurring pauses.

Note: When I speak about breathing exercises in my Check Engine Light classes, I'm often asked, "What about box breathing?" If you're unfamiliar, box breathing is a popular breathing technique that consists of a four-second inhale, a four-second hold, a four-second exhale, and another four-second hold. If at some point you want to experiment with this technique or another, by all means do so. I generally recommend the ratios above because six breaths per minute has a preponderance of research behind it.

Progressive Relaxation

Progressive relaxation is a tool that focuses your attention on your internal perception of your body (interoception) while you purposefully relax your muscles in a stepwise manner. You usually start at your feet and work your way up, as you will do for this exercise, but after you get the hang of it, you can do it in whatever order you want. Over time, you're free to tinker with it to find what works best for you.

Sit or lie down in a comfortable position. Choose a quiet space or wear noise-canceling headphones. If you try to do progressive relaxation in your living room just before dinner and your kids are running all over the house and your dog is barking, then this exercise probably won't work too well. (If you can truly relax while all of that is happening around you, you don't need this exercise.)

Set a timer for five minutes. Five minutes is the minimum, but up to ten minutes is acceptable. To fill ten minutes, you may have to repeat the exercise.

1. If you're not in a dark room, close your eyes. An eye mask can be helpful as well.

2. Focus your attention on your breathing for a few breaths. Feel the air moving in and out.

3. Bring your attention to your feet, ankles, and lower legs. For a few breaths, just notice them. Feel the temperature of your feet. Notice the blood flowing. Feel for any stiffness or discomfort. Inhale deeply, hold your breath, and now point your toes for three seconds. As you exhale, relax your feet and let them get heavy. Repeat this process once more, this time flexing your toes up toward your knees after the inhale.

4. Feel your breath again for one or two breaths.

5. Bring your attention to your lower legs and knees. For a few breaths, just notice them. Feel the blood flowing through them. Notice any stiffness or discomfort. Accept the sensations that are present. Inhale deeply, hold your breath, and now straighten your legs with effort. Create real tension! As you exhale, relax your legs and let them get heavier and heavier. Repeat this process once or twice.

6. Feel your breath again for one or two breaths. Imagine your body getting heavier and heavier.

7. Bring your attention to your hips and abdominals. For a few breaths, just notice the sensations in this area. Notice their temperature. Feel the blood flowing through them. Notice any stiffness or discomfort. Inhale deeply, hold your breath, and squeeze your butt and belly tight. As you exhale, let your belly soften and let your butt sink. Get heavy. Repeat this process once or twice.

8. Feel your breath again for one or two breaths. Imagine your body getting heavier and heavier.

9. Bring your attention to your arms and shoulders. For a few breaths, just notice them. Feel the blood flowing through them. Notice any stiffness or discomfort. Now inhale deeply, hold your breath, and squeeze your fists tightly while you push your shoulder blades back. As you exhale, relax your hands and let your arms and shoulders get heavy. Let them sink into the ground. Repeat this process once or twice.

10. Feel your breath again for one or two breaths. Feel how heavy you are now.

11. Bring your attention to your head and face. For a few breaths, just notice them. Feel the blood flowing through them. Notice any stiffness or discomfort. Now inhale deeply, hold your breath, and scowl and grit your teeth. As you exhale, let your face soften and let your head get heavy. Repeat this process once or twice.

12. Bring your attention once more to your breathing. Feel it soften as you get heavier and heavier.

13. Repeat the entire process or any section of it if you wish.

STARTING SURVEY

Answer the following questions based on the past week of your life.

	Never	Rarely	Sometimes	Often	Always
I have found it difficult to shake off negative thoughts and feelings.	○	○	○	○	○
I have felt upset.	○	○	○	○	○
I have felt anxious.	○	○	○	○	○
I have felt uneasy.	○	○	○	○	○
I have felt overwhelmed.	○	○	○	○	○

	Never	Rarely	Sometimes	Often	Always
I have been easily distracted.	○	○	○	○	○
My heart has been racing without physical exertion.	○	○	○	○	○
I have experienced shortness of breath without physical exertion.	○	○	○	○	○
My thoughts were negative.	○	○	○	○	○

On average, I fall at this level on the Stress Continuum:	○ Green	○ Yellow	○ Orange	○ Red

STRESS CONTINUUM			
GREEN Ready	**YELLOW** Reacting	**ORANGE** Injured	**RED** Critical
Healthy Sleep	Sleep Loss	Sleep Issues/ Nightmares	Insomnia
Healthy Personal Relationships	Distance from Others	Disengaged Relationships	Broken Relationships
Spiritual & Emotional Health	Change in Attitude	Feeling Trapped	Intrusive Thoughts
Physical Health	Fatigue	Exhausted	Anxiety & Panic
Emotionally Available	Avoidance Short Fuse	Physical Symptoms	Depression
Gratitude	Criticism	Emotional Numbness	Feeling Lost or Out of Control
Vitality	Lack of Motivation	Suffering	Thoughts of Suicide
Room for Complexity	Cutting Corners	Isolation	Blame
Sense of Mission	Loss of Creativity Loss of Interest	Burnout	Hopelessness

Adapted from Combat and Operational Stress First Aid by Laura McGladrey, ResponderAlliance.com

DAILY SURVEY

Take this survey at the end of each day during the experiment.

	Strongly disagree	Disagree	Neutral	Agree	Strongly agree
The exercises I performed today increased my awareness of my stress in my body.	O	O	O	O	O
The exercises helped reduce my stress.	O	O	O	O	O
The exercises helped improve my day.	O	O	O	O	O
The exercises energized me.	O	O	O	O	O
The exercises calmed my mind.	O	O	O	O	O
The exercises made me more resilient to daily stressors.	O	O	O	O	O
The exercises made me tired.	O	O	O	O	O
Describe any other insights you have gained from performing these exercises.					

ENDING SURVEY AND REFLECTION QUESTIONS

After completing the experiment, answer these questions to reflect on what you've learned. What changed? Why? What can you do next? Did something change that you didn't expect? All of these types of lessons and more as you engage!

Where are you on the Stress Continuum after fifteen days?	O Green	O Yellow	O Orange	O Red
What connections did you notice between the more objective KPIs (HRV, resting heart rate, etc.) and your internal sense of stress?				

	Strongly disagree	Disagree	Neutral	Agree	Strongly agree
The exercises gave me a new perspective on how my autonomic nervous system reflects my level of stress.	○	○	○	○	○
This experiment helped me make better sense of how my body reacts to stress.	○	○	○	○	○
I learned something important about my mind.	○	○	○	○	○
If so, briefly describe what you learned.					
This experiment helped me find indicators that I can put on my Performance Longevity Dashboard.	○	○	○	○	○
If so, what are they?					
I noticed connections to other categories in the M3 Model.	○	○	○	○	○
If so, what were they?					
I would recommend this experiment to a friend or family member.	○	○	○	○	○
Will anything you learned in this experiment affect how you approach this aspect of your performance longevity in the future? If so, what was it?					
Write a brief but specific statement describing something you learned that surprised you.					

Experiment #2: Emotional Well-Being

This experiment focuses on the effects that different types of writing practices may have on your emotional well-being. Writing is a way of making what's going on inside of you come out in a more concrete form so that you can see it right in front of you. When you are managing the complex landscape of your emotions, it can be difficult to stop spinning all of those plates so you can see what you're really dealing with. The practices in this experiment by no means offer the be-all, end-all when it comes to managing emotions, but they can help you become more aware of what's going on internally. Often, that's enough to get the ball rolling in the right direction.

Description

Run time: Fifteen days.

Using experiment indicators: The indicators for this experiment are the starting survey, daily survey, and ending survey and reflection questions provided. Take the daily survey before using the tool each day.

Using experiment tools: The tools for this experiment are Morning Pages and gratitude writing. At the start of each day, preferably within ninety minutes of waking, perform the intervention of your choice at a consistent time, adjusting as needed, and stick with it for at least five days.

Indicators

The indicators for this experiment are the starting survey and daily survey provided after the tools.

Tools

Morning Pages

Morning Pages is an exercise originally developed by Julia Cameron to help artists tap into deeper creativity, but it is applicable in the realm of emotional well-being, too. The instructions are to handwrite three pages on paper. Pay no attention to sentence structure, spelling, or grammar. Keep your writing utensil on the page and simply allow whatever comes through to land on the page. What you write does not need to be a cathartic diary or journal, but at times it might be. Just write whatever comes out—poems, phrases, quotes, whatever. Let it flow.

Write these pages first thing in the morning every day for at least five days. I suggest keeping a notebook and pen or pencil in the same exact place for this purpose. I do realize that this much writing can be a lot, so one to three pages, which should take you between ten and thirty minutes to complete, is a nice goal to start with. Remember, there's no specific subject matter. Just write.

Gratitude Writing

Gratitude writing is all about finding the good things in life, no matter how small. This tool differs from Morning Pages in that you cover a specific subject. Gratitude writing has been shown to be an effective tool in the field of psychology. It may help some people reduce stress and gain perspective.

This brief questionnaire asks short-answer questions that relate to gratitude. Spend five to ten minutes each day thinking deeply about these questions, and be honest with your answers.

I am thankful for _____ [name a person, place, or thing].

Without it/them, I would be _____. Answer with one or two complete sentences. Think!

Having it/them helps me _____. Answer with one or two complete sentences.

Extra credit: If your thing is a person, tell them that you're grateful for them and why. If it's a place or thing, tell somebody that you're grateful for it. If you're not sure who to tell, say it out loud to yourself.

STARTING SURVEY

Answer the following questions based on the past week of your life.

Are you aware of how your emotions and physical state influence each other? If so, how?

_____

_____

Give examples of how something physical alters your mood as well as an example of how your mood alters your emotional state.

_____

_____

How do you typically respond to stress?

_____

_____

When I feel stressed, my initial reaction is to (choose one):	○ Take immediate action	○ Avoid the situation
	○ Become overwhelmed	○ Process it over time

Provide an example of a recent stressful situation and how you handled it.

_____

_____

When you feel emotionally off, what do you typically do to reset? List any strategies or habits you use, such as movement, writing, talking to someone, or simply waiting for it to pass.

_____

_____

MIND EXPERIMENTS

Do you intentionally set aside time to think about your emotions? If so, how much time do you spend, and in what form do you reflect (e.g., journaling, meditation, informal reflection)? If not, do you feel like your emotions still influence your daily choices?

_____

_____

DAILY SURVEY

Take this survey at the end of each day during the experiment.

My general mood today was:					

	Strongly disagree	Disagree	Neutral	Agree	Strongly agree
I felt motivated.	○	○	○	○	○
I felt low in energy.	○	○	○	○	○
My body felt slow and heavy.	○	○	○	○	○
My body felt light.	○	○	○	○	○
I had lots of energy.	○	○	○	○	○
I felt ready to meet challenges as they arose.	○	○	○	○	○
I got upset today.	○	○	○	○	○
If I got upset, it took a while for me to calm down.	○	○	○	○	○
The exercise helped me identify my feelings more clearly.	○	○	○	○	○
The exercise helped me change how I was feeling if I wanted to.	○	○	○	○	○

ENDING SURVEY AND REFLECTION QUESTIONS

Answer these questions after completing the experiment to reflect on what you've learned. What changed? Why? What can you do next? Did something change that you didn't expect? All of these types of lessons and more as you engage!

	Strongly disagree	Disagree	Neutral	Agree	Strongly agree
The exercises gave me a new perspective on my emotions.	○	○	○	○	○
If so, briefly describe what you learned.					
I learned something important about my mind.	○	○	○	○	○
If so, briefly describe what you learned.					
This experiment helped me find indicators that I can put on my Performance Longevity Dashboard.	○	○	○	○	○
If so, what are they?					
I noticed connections to other categories in the M3 Model.	○	○	○	○	○
If so, what were they?					
I would recommend this experiment to a friend or family member.	○	○	○	○	○
Will anything you learned in this experiment affect how you approach this aspect of your performance longevity in the future? If so, what was it?					

	Strongly disagree	Disagree	Neutral	Agree	Strongly agree
As a result of doing this experiment, I am more likely to continue experimenting.	○	○	○	○	○
What would you want to try next?					
Write a brief but specific statement describing something you learned that surprised you.					

Experiment #3: Cognitive Powers

This final potential experiment in the MIND category can help you tune some fundamental cognitive powers: the ability to purposefully focus and disperse attention. These two functions have been the study of many meditation and thought development practices. The simple tools offered in this experiment are, as with all of the tools offered in this book, only meant as starting places for building your toolkit. See how they work for you, keep what you like, discard what you don't, and then keep searching!

Description

Run time: Fifteen days.

Using experiment indicators: The indicators for this experiment are the starting survey, daily survey, and ending survey and reflection questions provided. Take the daily survey before using the tool each day.

Using experiment tools: The interventions for this experiment, reverie and deep focus, take between thirty and sixty minutes because they are cognitive tools. Be sure to plan accordingly. The best time to use these tools is within ninety minutes of waking, before the weight of the day settles on your brain. However, life doesn't perfectly align with these experiments, so whatever time you find for the tools, be consistent.

Indicators

The indicators for this experiment are the starting survey and daily survey provided after the tools.

Tools

Reverie

Reverie is the simple act of letting your mind wander without any deliberate focus. No technology. No screens, no phones, no watches or gadgets of any kind. No music, no books, no magazines. No socializing. No meditating or relaxation exercises. Reverie is directly connected to the "Rest Is Not Idleness" section of Chapter 4.

Each day, you'll set aside ten to thirty minutes for reverie. This could be during your work commute, while sitting on your porch, or before or after your lunch break—it doesn't matter. What is important is that you just let your mind wander during that time period and think about whatever it wants to.

STARTING SURVEY: REVERIE

Answer the following questions based on the past week of your life.

	Never	Rarely	Sometimes	Often	Always
I dwell on repetitive thoughts that cause me distress.	○	○	○	○	○
Repetitive thoughts are a distraction when I'm spending time with family or friends.	○	○	○	○	○
I obsess over problems in my life.	○	○	○	○	○
I have trouble letting things go.	○	○	○	○	○
I have a hard time totally relaxing.	○	○	○	○	○

ENDING SURVEY AND REFLECTION QUESTIONS: REVERIE

Answer these questions after completing the experiment.

	Never	Rarely	Sometimes	Often	Always
I dwell on repetitive thoughts that cause me distress.	○	○	○	○	○
Repetitive thoughts are a distraction when I'm spending time with family or friends.	○	○	○	○	○
I obsess over problems in my life.	○	○	○	○	○
I have trouble letting things go.	○	○	○	○	○
I have a hard time totally relaxing.	○	○	○	○	○

	Strongly disagree	Disagree	Neutral	Agree	Strongly agree
In general, my awareness of my thought patterns has changed for the better.	○	○	○	○	○
This experiment helped me make better sense of my cognitive abilities.	○	○	○	○	○
If so, how?					
I learned something important about my mind.	○	○	○	○	○
If so, briefly describe what you learned.					

What indicators have you learned about that you can put on your Performance Longevity Dashboard? How will you keep using these tools? Are there new tools you might try?					
	Strongly disagree	**Disagree**	**Neutral**	**Agree**	**Strongly agree**
I noticed connections to other categories in the M3 Model.	○	○	○	○	○
If so, what were they?					
I would recommend this experiment to a friend or family member.	○	○	○	○	○
Will anything you learned in this experiment affect how you approach this aspect of your performance longevity in the future? If so, what was it?					
Write a brief but specific statement describing something you learned that surprised you.					

Deep Focus

Focusing the mind intently on a singular effort and for extended periods is a valuable skill no matter what job you have or what hobbies you enjoy. Learning to focus your attention and sustain that focus can help make you more productive and efficient when trying to accomplish tasks, learning new things, or just being a more present friend or partner. Focusing attention is a skill that through practice can enrich your life in the short and long term. Use it or lose it!

Each day, you'll set aside fifteen to sixty minutes for focus. During this time, you will remove all distractions—no screens, no music, no white noise. Just you and your brain. Find a singular item to focus on. Read a book, write in a journal, or practice a skill, like playing the guitar or crocheting. Focus all of your attention on that thing and nothing else. Make sure that if you live with other people, they know what you're doing, or else it may cause a social issue. Better yet, invite their participation.

STARTING SURVEY: DEEP FOCUS

Answer the following questions based on the past week of your life.

	Strongly disagree	Disagree	Neutral	Agree	Strongly agree
I'm easily distracted when I try to focus on a single thing.	○	○	○	○	○
Give an example of a situation where you get distracted.					
I'm not as productive as I want to be.	○	○	○	○	○
What happens when you feel unproductive?					

	Never	Rarely	Sometimes	Often	Always
When I get distracted, it's difficult to get back on track.	○	○	○	○	○
I use a substance to help keep me focused.	○	○	○	○	○
If so, what is it?					

DAILY SURVEY

Use this survey for both Reverie and Deep Focus.

How much time were you able to commit to the experiment today?	15 minutes	15–30 minutes	30–45 minutes	45–60 minutes	60+ minutes

	Strongly disagree	Disagree	Neutral	Agree	Strongly agree
(Skip if doing reverie experiment) I could easily focus during the focus time.	○	○	○	○	○
(Skip if doing focus experiment) I could easily allow my mind to wander without a specific task.	○	○	○	○	○
I felt frustrated when doing this experiment.	○	○	○	○	○

Frustration is a sign of:	Total and utter failure	Learning	Me not getting what I want

If I stick with this practice, I'll get better.	Strongly disagree	Disagree	Neutral	Agree	Strongly agree

My screen time today was _____ hours.	0–3	3–5	5+

	Strongly disagree	Disagree	Neutral	Agree	Strongly agree
I felt an increase in mental energy.	○	○	○	○	○
I felt a decrease in mental energy.	○	○	○	○	○

ENDING SURVEY AND REFLECTION QUESTIONS

Answer these questions after completing the experiment (either Reverie or Deep Focus) to reflect on what you've learned. What changed? Why? What can you do next? Did something change that you didn't expect? All of these types of lessons and more as you engage!

	Strongly disagree	Disagree	Neutral	Agree	Strongly agree
I have more mental energy throughout the day.	○	○	○	○	○
I feel less distracted during the focus time.	○	○	○	○	○
I am able to focus on tasks outside of the focus exercise more easily.	○	○	○	○	○
I feel more productive.	○	○	○	○	○
This experiment increased my confidence in my ability to train my brain.	○	○	○	○	○
I catch myself earlier when I'm getting distracted.	○	○	○	○	○
I can refocus my attention more easily.	○	○	○	○	○
The exercises gave me a new perspective on my mind.	○	○	○	○	○
If so, briefly describe what you learned.					
This experiment helped me make better sense of my cognitive abilities.	○	○	○	○	○
If so, briefly describe what you learned.					

	Strongly disagree	Disagree	Neutral	Agree	Strongly agree
I learned something important about my mind in this experiment.	○	○	○	○	○
If so, briefly describe what you learned.					
This experiment helped me find indicators that I can put on my Performance Longevity Dashboard.	○	○	○	○	○
If so, what are they?					
I noticed connections to other categories in the M3 Model.	○	○	○	○	○
If so, what were they?					
I would recommend this experiment to a friend or family member.	○	○	○	○	○
Will anything you learned in this experiment affect how you approach this aspect of your performance longevity in the future? If so, what was it?					
Write a brief but specific statement describing something you learned that surprised you.					

MVMT EXPERIMENTS

Experiment #1: Isometrics

Isometric strength and endurance are fundamental qualities of fitness. As well as being safe forms of strength training, they are some of the most challenging and far-reaching types of exercise when it comes to benefits. They're used in everything from athletic conditioning and martial arts to rehabilitative settings.

As always, if you're unsure whether a movement pattern or metric is safe for you, ask a trusted healthcare provider. (Outsource!) Just as with the previous experiment, it is important to learn the difference between injury potential and plain old discomfort. In the case of movement, one stunts your progress and the other catalyzes it.

Description

Run time: Fifteen days.

Using experiment indicators: The indicators for this experiment are time under tension and blood pressure. Choose one of these as your primary indicator and measure it daily at the same time of day. You may use both indicators if you want, but maintain a single primary indicator for the entirety of the experiment. For consistency, take measurements first thing in the morning before consuming caffeine or other stimulants and before using the tool.

Using experiment tools: The tools for this experiment are horse stance, plank, and wall push. Perform the intervention of your choice at a consistent time, adjusting as needed, and stick with it for at least five days.

Indicators

Time Under Tension

1. Choose a movement pattern from the menu under Tools: horse stance, plank, or wall push.

2. Hold the position with maximum effort until you reach near failure—just before muscle fatigue causes you to collapse.

3. Rest between holds for at least two minutes, but no more than five minutes, before repeating the exercise.

4. Repeat the hold to near failure a second time.

5. Record your total hold time (in minutes and seconds) for both attempts—this is your first measurement.

6. On the last day of the experiment, repeat the process and compare your new times to your initial results.

Blood Pressure

What the heck does blood pressure have to do with isometric exercise? Let's find out. Remember, MIND, MVMT, and MTTR interact all the time.

You'll take your blood pressure each day before doing the exercise. Isometric contractions can temporarily raise blood pressure during the effort, so a resting measurement beforehand gives you the most consistent and useful data. If you want to measure after the exercise as well, you can—but the number that matters most for tracking change is the one you take before you start, after a few minutes of rest.

Each day, repeat your isometric exercise, and monitor how your blood pressure responds over time.

Tools

Pick the horse stance, plank, or wall push as your movement pattern of focus for this experiment. Each day, you will perform three or four holds in your chosen movement at 40 to 60 percent of your total time from day 1. So, if you held for 2 minutes, or 120 seconds, that would be a 48- to 72-second hold repeated three or four times. These are general recommendations. I'm not there with you, so if you need to shorten the time to maintain good standards (formal movement!), then do so. Likewise, if you need to adjust it upward for more of a challenge, you can, as long as you can maintain the standard of execution for each exercise.

Horse Stance

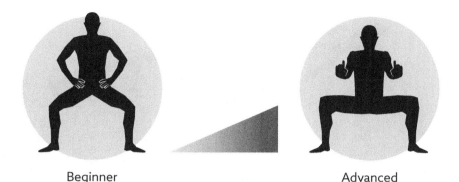

Beginner   Advanced

Setup and Alignment:

- Feet: Flat on the ground, turned slightly outward, wider than shoulder width apart

- Posture: Keep head, shoulders, and hips stacked vertically

- Arms: For beginner, hands on hips; for intermediate/advanced, extend arms forward, to the sides, or in guard position

- Knees: Bend to a comfortable depth, ideally working toward thighs parallel to the ground (~90°) and keeping knees aligned with toes— avoid letting them collapse inward or shift too far outward

Breathing Cues:

- Inhale through the nose while setting your posture.

- Exhale slowly through the nose or mouth as you settle into the stance.

- Maintain steady, rhythmic breathing throughout the hold—don't hold your breath.

- Focus on core engagement during each exhale to stabilize the spine and support alignment.

Plank

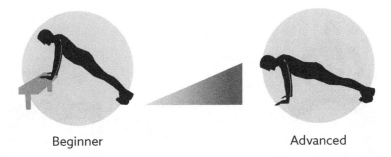

Beginner   Advanced

Setup and Alignment:

- Arms: Straight and active, with shoulders stacked directly over wrists

- Hands: Press firmly into the ground or elevated surface, creating full-body tension

- Legs: Extended straight back, feet hip width apart

- Core and glutes: Engage abdominals, glutes, and legs to maintain a rigid, aligned position

- Spine: Keep a neutral neck and spine—avoid sagging or arching

Support Options (Regression):

- Use a stable elevated surface (such as a box, couch, chair, or stair) to reduce intensity while maintaining form.

- As strength improves, gradually lower the angle to increase the challenge.

Breathing Cues:

- Breathe slowly and smoothly through the nose or mouth.

- Avoid breath holding—each exhale can help reinforce full-body tension.

Coaching Tip: Think of your body as a solid plank from head to heels—no sagging in the hips, no lifting of the butt. Actively push the ground away and imagine drawing your ribs toward your pelvis to build tension throughout your body.

Wall Push

Bear Crawl Push (Wall Crawl Version)

A ground-based wall push emphasizing core stability, full-body alignment, and tension.

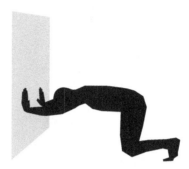

Setup and Alignment:

- Hands pressed into the wall at shoulder height
- Arms fully extended, with wrists, elbows, shoulders, torso, and hips aligned
- Knees, hips, and ankles bent to approximately 90 degrees
- Toes tucked, heels slightly elevated

Execution:

- Actively press into the wall as if attempting to push it away.
- Generate force from the legs, through the hips and core, into the arms.
- Maintain full-body tension and a neutral spine alignment.
- Breathe slowly and smoothly.

Standing Wall Push

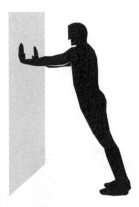

A standing version that encourages full kinetic chain engagement and postural alignment.

Setup and Alignment:

- Staggered stance (natural step length), feet roughly hip to shoulder width apart
- Arms extended forward, hands pressed against a wall at shoulder height

Execution:

- Actively drive into the wall using force from your rear leg through the torso and into the arms.
- Keep your arms straight and active, shoulders packed.
- Maintain upright posture and abdominal engagement.

STARTING SURVEY

Answer the following questions based on the past week of your life.

	Strongly disagree	Disagree	Neutral	Agree	Strongly agree
If my body is uncomfortable, something is wrong. (Think about your answer. Does your behavior reflect this response?)	○	○	○	○	○
I enjoy physical effort.	○	○	○	○	○
I am strong.	○	○	○	○	○
Physical challenges help my body.	○	○	○	○	○
I can overcome physical challenges.	○	○	○	○	○

DAILY SURVEY

Take this survey at the end of each day during the experiment.

	Strongly disagree	Disagree	Neutral	Agree	Strongly agree
I went to bed on time last night.	○	○	○	○	○

I drank _____ alcoholic drinks yesterday.	○ 0	○ 1–2	○ 2–4	○ 5+

I ate within _____ minutes of bedtime.	○ 30–60	○ 60–90	○ 90–120	○ 120+

	Strongly disagree	Disagree	Neutral	Agree	Strongly agree
I had a stressful day yesterday.	○	○	○	○	○
I woke up energized.	○	○	○	○	○
I woke up motivated to do this exercise.	○	○	○	○	○

I felt _____ today.	○ Very weak	○ Somewhat weak	○ Somewhat strong	○ Strong	○ Very strong

	Strongly disagree	Disagree	Neutral	Agree	Strongly agree
I had to use more mental effort to do the exercise.	○	○	○	○	○
My legs/arms burned like crazy during the exercise.	○	○	○	○	○
Controlling my breathing was easier.	○	○	○	○	○

Compared to yesterday, my self-talk during the exercise was more:	○ Negative	○ Neutral	○ Positive

	Strongly disagree	Disagree	Neutral	Agree	Strongly agree
This exercise makes me feel stronger.	○	○	○	○	○
This exercise is building my confidence.	○	○	○	○	○
How did performing this exercise affect the rest of your day?	_____				

ENDING SURVEY AND REFLECTION QUESTIONS

Answer these questions after completing the experiment to reflect on what you've learned. What changed? Why? What can you do next? Did something change that you didn't expect? All of these types of lessons and more as you engage!

	Strongly disagree	Disagree	Neutral	Agree	Strongly agree
Isometric exercise will continue to be a part of my formal movement practice.	○	○	○	○	○
This experiment helped me make better sense of the sensations in my body.	○	○	○	○	○
If so, how?					
I learned something important about how my body moves.	○	○	○	○	○
If so, briefly describe what you learned.					
This experiment helped me find indicators that I can put on my Performance Longevity Dashboard.	○	○	○	○	○
If so, what are they?					
I noticed connections to other categories in the M3 Model.	○	○	○	○	○
If so, what were they?					

Will anything you learned in this experiment affect how you approach this aspect of your performance longevity in the future? If so, what was it?					
	Strongly disagree	Disagree	Neutral	Agree	Strongly agree
I would recommend this experiment to a friend or family member.	◯	◯	◯	◯	◯
As a result of doing this experiment, I am more likely to continue experimenting.	◯	◯	◯	◯	◯
What other experiments could you do? Write down a few examples for later reference.					
Write a brief but specific statement describing something you learned that surprised you.					

Experiment #2: Balance, Daniel-San

Balance is, technically speaking, the ability to keep your center of mass over your base of support. Not so technically speaking, it's what keeps you from falling ass over teakettle while you do things. If you're standing still with both feet on the ground, that's your torso over your feet. Balance can include both static variations, as in simply standing in place on one leg, and more dynamic variations, where there are transitions between multiple positions that require fluid starting and stopping over a base of support.

Balance is another movement capability that can steadily slip out of your grasp without some form of regular touchpoint. The human body is built for organic efficiency, so it is often the case that we don't realize our balance stinks until life exposes it through some less-than-preferable way. Maintaining some standard of balance through the use of simple exercises can be helpful.

For this experiment, you'll do graduated variations of simple exercises that involve standing on one foot. You may find some variations more challenging than others, and for different reasons. A host of factors affect our ability to orient ourselves in the space around us. As you use the daily markers of movement, remember not to fixate on a thought of good/better/best. As discussed, some standardization is important, but even more important is to know what shifts you're experiencing from day to day, month to month, and year to year.

You can do this experiment as a seasonal focus and/or include some part of it in a daily routine you already have. I use the leg circle variation as part of my daily function check along with Sun Salutation. The exercise serves not only as a great way to preserve my movement abilities, but also as a daily evaluation tool for how my body is doing in general. One thing I've noticed is that my balance is greatly correlated with my overall neurocognitive sharpness.

Description

Run time: Fifteen days.

Using experiment indicators: Start with the static hold balance test and, if you pass, move on to the single-leg reach dynamic balance test. Repeat the single-leg reach at the end of the experiment to track your improvement. For consistency, take measurements first thing in the morning before consuming caffeine or other stimulants. Answer the daily survey before using the tool each day.

Using experiment tools: Here, the tools are the same as the indicators, with one addition: one-legged hip circles. Perform the intervention at a consistent time, adjusting as needed, and stick with it for at least five days. Start with the static hold and, if you can, progress to the single-leg reach and one-legged hip circles as directed on the following pages.

Indicators

Perform each exercise barefoot or in socks, on a level floor free of obstacles.

Static Hold (Balance Test):

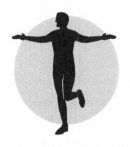

1. Stand on one leg with the other leg bent and lifted as high as possible.

2. Extend your arms to the sides and hold for as long as you can.

3. Repeat on the other leg.

4. If you can hold for more than thirty seconds on each leg, move on to the next indicator.

Single-Leg Reach (Dynamic Balance Test):

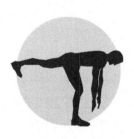

1. Stand on one foot, pressing firmly into the ground with your support leg and foot.

2. Lift the other foot and extend it behind you as you reach your arms as far forward as possible, touching the floor if possible.

3. Perform twice on each leg.

Key Performance Indicators:

- Measure the distance you can reach from the big toe of your balancing leg. (Place a piece of tape at your big toe, then another at your max reach; enlist a helper if you can.)

- Observe how much your support leg bends to allow the reach.

- If you can't touch the floor without losing your balance, skip this test and stick with the static hold.

Tools

Some tools double as indicators, which means that performing them helps improve the very thing you're measuring. Your ability to stand on one leg for thirty seconds determines which tool(s) you will use.

- If you cannot hold a single-leg stance for thirty seconds, stick with the Static Hold.

- If you can hold for thirty-plus seconds for at least five consecutive days, progress to the next two tools.

Perform these balance and coordination exercises first thing in the morning, before consuming caffeine or other stimulants. Immediately after, fill out the daily survey or at least review the questions and reflect. This is a MVMT experiment, but your goal is to connect insights across MIND, MVMT, and MTTR.

Guidelines for all three tools:

- Breathe deeply and evenly through your nose.

- Coordinate your inhales and exhales with your movement.

- Don't rush—focus on slow, controlled execution.

Static Hold

Perform the movement as described under "Indicators." Do two or three sets of holding on one leg for as long as you can, up to thirty seconds per side. Once you can consistently hold for thirty or more seconds for five straight days, move on to one of the next two tools.

Single-Leg Reach (For Those Who Pass the Static Hold Test)

Perform the movement as described under "Indicators." Do five to ten reps on each leg, doing two or three sets daily.

Use the same form as the indicator test, but don't measure—focus on control.

One-Legged Hip Circles (Advanced Coordination and Strength)

Perform three to five reps on each leg, doing two sets daily. Each full rotation is one rep.

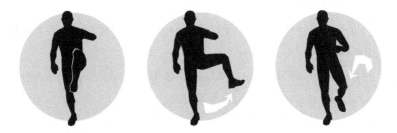

1. Lift your bent leg in front of you as high as possible.

2. Rotate your foot outward, as if stepping backward over a stool.

3. Extend your leg straight back, then bring it forward without touching the ground.

STARTING SURVEY

Answer the following questions based on the past week of your life.

	Strongly disagree	Disagree	Neutral	Agree	Strongly agree
I have great balance.	○	○	○	○	○
I was surprised by my results in the initial experiment test.	○	○	○	○	○
I have great control over my body.	○	○	○	○	○
My body can get better at things if I practice.	○	○	○	○	○
My stress levels affect my ability to move well.	○	○	○	○	○
I can focus in spite of stress.	○	○	○	○	○

DAILY SURVEY

Take this survey at the end of each day during the experiment.

	Strongly disagree	Disagree	Neutral	Agree	Strongly agree
I slept well last night.	○	○	○	○	○
I felt well rested this morning.	○	○	○	○	○
I felt stressed today.	○	○	○	○	○
My movement felt smooth.	○	○	○	○	○
My breathing felt smooth.	○	○	○	○	○
I had trouble focusing my mind during the exercises.	○	○	○	○	○
I was aware of noise (excessive tension or wobbling) during the exercises.	○	○	○	○	○
If so, why do you think that is?					
How has that changed since yesterday? Or over the last couple of days?					
Have you noticed any correlation between changes in your MVMT and changes in MIND or MTTR? If so, what are they?					

ENDING SURVEY AND REFLECTION QUESTIONS

Answer these questions after completing the experiment to reflect on what you've learned. What changed? Why? What can you do next? Did something change that you didn't expect? All of these types of lessons and more as you engage!

	Strongly disagree	Disagree	Neutral	Agree	Strongly agree
I have great balance.	○	○	○	○	○
I was surprised by my results in the initial experiment test.	○	○	○	○	○
I have great control over my body.	○	○	○	○	○
My body can get better at things if I practice.	○	○	○	○	○
My stress levels affect my ability to move well.	○	○	○	○	○
I can focus in spite of stress.	○	○	○	○	○
This experiment helped me make better sense of the sensations in my body.	○	○	○	○	○
If so, how?					
I learned something important about how my body moves.	○	○	○	○	○
If so, briefly describe what you learned.					
This experiment helped me find indicators that I can put on my Performance Longevity Dashboard.	○	○	○	○	○
If so, what are they?					

	Strongly disagree	Disagree	Neutral	Agree	Strongly agree
I noticed connections to other categories in the M3 Model.	○	○	○	○	○
If so, what were they?					
Will anything you learned in this experiment affect how you approach this aspect of your Performance Longevity in the future? If so, what was it?					
I would recommend this experiment to a friend or family member.	○	○	○	○	○
As a result of doing this experiment, I am more likely to continue experimenting.	○	○	○	○	○
What other experiments could you do? Write down a few examples for later reference.					
Write a brief but specific statement describing something you learned that surprised you.					

Experiment #3: Sun Salutation

The Sun Salutation experiment is unique in its format compared to the other two MVMT experiments. While it does use metrics that could be considered somewhat objective, such as comparing range of motion in a particular pose, this experiment also offers some subjective metrics that are equally important. Those refer to the mood words that I discussed in Chapter 5. This subjectivity may be challenging initially for you dyed-in-the-wool Engineers. Those of you who are more of the Intuitive ilk will feel right at home.

While I hope you do enjoy some improvement in your ability to move freely and smoothly, that's not the only outcome I have in mind for this experiment. The bigger picture here is to see not only how your movement choices affect trends and patterns in your ability to move, but how *all* aspects of MIND, MVMT, and MTTR may affect your experience of your body over time.

This sequence provides insight into your daily movement capacity. For this experiment, you'll have options: perform the full sequence or isolate specific movements based on time, ability, or comfort. The pictograph outlines both approaches. Ideally, you'll complete the full sequence, but modifications are valid if needed.

Proceed with care and consult a medical professional if necessary. That said, challenge drives improvement. If no medical condition prohibits your movement, test your limits—sometimes avoidance signals an underlying issue.

Whether you do the entire sequence or just a portion of it, this exercise should take between one and ten minutes each day. I like to do it while my coffee is brewing. Take note of how many times you are performing it as you reflect on changes in the metrics you use to measure your movement. During this particular experiment, do the same number of cycles over the course of five-plus days. Feel free to add or subtract for a new period of experimentation, but try to keep it standardized initially for the purpose of fair comparison.

Description

Run time: Fifteen days.

Using experiment indicators: The indicators for this experiment are a little different from the others. Be sure to read the following paragraphs carefully so you know what to look for.

First, there's a survey that you'll take every day. The purpose of the survey is to help you not only reflect on day-to-day changes in how your body is moving but also connect how well your body is moving physically with other aspects of your behavior that you may not normally connect with movement—for example, how the previous night or two of sleep may have affected your movement quality.

Second, there are movement checkpoints that are represented as poses in each phase of the Sun Salutation. The focus points for the poses are displayed in the pictographs on the following pages. If you choose to single out a particular pose for this experiment, simply repeat that pose ten to fifteen times.

Using experiment tools: For this experiment, the tools are pose repetition and contract/relax stretching. These are done in an integrated fashion and are not performed separately from daily Sun Salutations.

Indicators

This experiment is a little different because the "tool" is in the form of Sun Salutation. Perform the entire sequence of postures (or a portion of it) for five to fifteen minutes at a consistent time each day, adjusting as needed.

Repeat the steps for each position for the given number of repetitions, actively coordinating your breath and motion and moving with focus and intent. On each rep, try to breathe slower, smoother, and more evenly and improve the coordination of your breath with your motion.

Tools

Pose Repetition

 Pose repetition is exactly what it sounds like. If you find a pose in the sequence that needs extra attention, simply go in and out of that pose three to five times. Don't just check the box, though. Move with intention and breathe smoothly and deeply. If you're doing just a portion of the Sun Salutation sequence for this experiment, then you'll perform ten to fifteen total repetitions of that pose.

Contract/Relax

  Contract/relax is a form of stretching that uses isometric contraction during stretches to elicit an improvement in movement quality and sometimes quantity, too. Many times, restrictions in motion are attributable to the nervous system putting the hand brake on movements you don't use. By using contract/relax and then moving in and out of shapes, you can improve not only your access to motion but also your relationship with the changing conditions of your neuromuscular system.

One way this shows up for me personally is in forward bends. This pose has always been particularly challenging for me, even when I'm at my most flexible. When I do contract/relax stretching during Sun Salutation, it's not just about going farther down in the forward bend. It's also an opportunity to see how my nervous system responds to this input. When I'm well rested, a bit of contract/relax goes a long way. When I'm fatigued or undernourished, not so much.

In short, contract/relax is another tool to affect your quantity and quality of movement, but also a way to become more attuned to your own body.

POSITION 1

Do 5–10 repetitions with FOCUS and INTENT.

 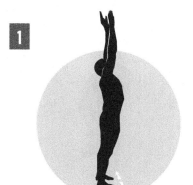

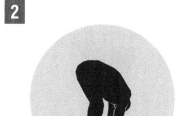

Inhale, reaching your arms overhead.

Actively press your hands and feet away from each other.

Exhale slowly while bending forward.

Use your abdominals to pull yourself forward as you reach for the ground.

Allow your knees to bend and your back to round slightly if needed.

1

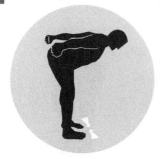

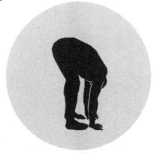 **2**

1

Inhale and hold for 2–3 seconds.

Stiffen a straight back.

Reach your arms back and your head forward while squeezing your feet toward each other.

GET TIGHT!

2

Slowly bend forward as you exhale.

Use your abdominals to pull yourself forward as you reach for the ground.

Allow your knees to bend and your back to round slightly if needed.

Take 3–5 breaths in the forward bend.

Repeat 2 or 3 times.

POSITION 2

1

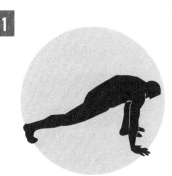

2

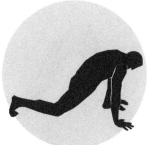

Press your hands and front foot into the ground.

Press hard through your back heel into a straight knee.

Squeeze your butt cheek tight.

Continue to press into the ground with your upper body.

Drop your knee slowly to the ground.

Press your leg straight again with intent.

Push through your heel with a strong, straight leg.

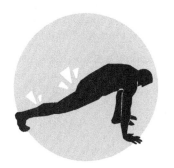

Inhale, then hold for 2–3 seconds.

Squeeze both legs and your butt tight.

Exhale and stop squeezing.

Look for ease and space in the shape.

Take 3–5 breaths in the shape.

Repeat 2 or 3 times.

POSITION 3

Do 5–10 repetitions with FOCUS and INTENT.

1

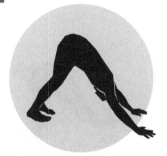

Press into the ground through spread fingers and straight arms.

Push your hands and hips away from each other.

A slight knee bend is okay.

Allow your heels to drop.

2

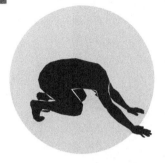

Inhale.

Bend your knees and allow them to drop toward the floor.

Exhale.

Actively press into down dog.

Look for small improvements each time you repeat.

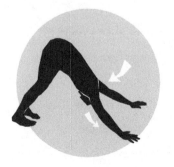

Inhale, hold, press your locked arms and shoulder blades actively toward the ground while moving your head toward your feet.

Exhale slowly, holding the shape but backing off the pressure. Spread your fingers and allow your armpits to sink toward the floor.

POSITION 4

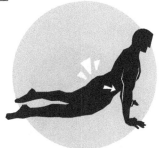

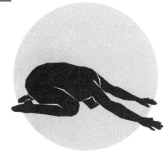

Inhale.

Press into the ground through spread fingers and straight arms.

Actively press your hips forward and squeeze your butt.

Keep your head up and look forward.

Exhale.

Sit your butt back to your heels.

Reach your hands actively away from your butt.

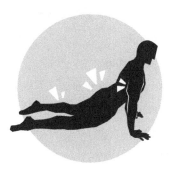

1. Inhale, then hold for 2–3 seconds.

   Hold the upward dog position while ramping up total body tension.

   Squeeze your arms, butt, and legs tight!

2. Exhale slowly.

   Back off tension.

   Look for new space and ease.

   Take 3–5 breaths in the shape.

   Repeat 2 or 3 times.

POSITION 5

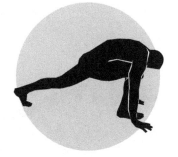 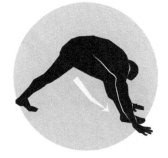

Inhale.

Press your hands and front foot into the ground.

Press hard through your back heel into a straight knee.

Squeeze your butt cheek tight.

Exhale.

Actively extend your front leg.

Press your front foot into the ground. A bend in the knee is okay.

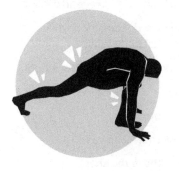

Inhale, then hold for 2–3 seconds.

Squeeze both your front and back leg tight.

Squeeze your butt tight.

Exhale and stop squeezing.

Look for ease and space in the shape.

Take 3–5 breaths in the shape.

Repeat 2 or 3 times.

POSITION 6

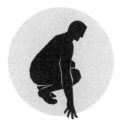

1

Inhale.

Bend your knees and come up onto your toes.

Keep your back straight.

Use active arms for support.

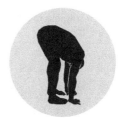

2

Press your heels and hands into the ground.

Allow your knees to bend and your back to round, but press your hips away from your feet.

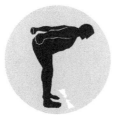

1

Inhale and hold for 2–3 seconds.

Stiffen a straight back.

Reach your arms back and your head forward.

Squeeze your feet toward each other.

GET TIGHT!

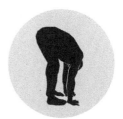

2

Slowly bend forward as you exhale.

Use your abdominals to pull yourself forward as you reach for the ground.

Allow your knees to bend and your back to round slightly if needed.

Take 3-5 breaths in forward bend.

Repeat 2 or 3 times.

Answer the following questions based on the past week of your life.

	Never	Rarely	Sometimes	Often	Always
I experience pain in my body.	○	○	○	○	○
I have areas of stiffness that I want to alleviate.	○	○	○	○	○
If so, where are they? What do you imagine will happen if you change them?					
I had an injury that affects my ability to move well.	○	○	○	○	○

Prior to this experiment, I devoted ____ days per week to formal movement.	○ 0	○ 1-3	○ 4+

	Never	Rarely	Sometimes	Often	Always
I practice some sort of formal movement.	○	○	○	○	○
If so, what is it? Can you describe the standards?					

DAILY SURVEY

Each day, fill out this survey after you perform the Sun Salutation sequence and then retest the metric of your choice. It should only take a minute or so.

	Strongly disagree	Disagree	Neutral	Agree	Strongly agree
I felt motivated to perform the exercise today.	○	○	○	○	○
I woke up full of energy.	○	○	○	○	○
I felt stiff and creaky.	○	○	○	○	○
I felt like a well-oiled machine.	○	○	○	○	○
I was in pain this morning.	○	○	○	○	○

After doing the exercise, my pain was:	○ The same	○ Better	○ Worse

The exercise helped me identify an area of stiffness in my body.	○	○	○	○	○
If so, what was it?	_____ _____				
The exercise relieved some stiffness in my body.	○	○	○	○	○

After doing the exercise, I felt:	Worse	Exactly the same	Somewhat better	Much better	Reborn
	○	○	○	○	○

I saw a change in the metric I used after I did the exercise.	○	○	○	○	○
If so, what changed?	_____ _____				

	Strongly disagree	Disagree	Neutral	Agree	Strongly agree
The amount of motion improved as I continued the exercise.	O	O	O	O	O
The quality of my movement feels better.	O	O	O	O	O
If applicable, what happened yesterday that may have negatively affected your movement? Think about all three categories of the M3 Model.					
If applicable, what happened yesterday that may have positively affected your movement? Think about all three categories of the M3 Model.					

ENDING SURVEY AND REFLECTION QUESTIONS

Answer these questions after completing the experiment to reflect on what you've learned. What changed? Why? What can you do next? Did something change that you didn't expect? All of these types of lessons and more as you engage!

	Strongly disagree	Disagree	Neutral	Agree	Strongly agree
Sun Salutation (or some part of it) will continue to be a part of my morning routine.	O	O	O	O	O
This experiment helped me make better sense of the sensations in my body.	O	O	O	O	O
I learned something important about how my body moves.	O	O	O	O	O
If so, briefly describe what you learned.					

MTTR EXPERIMENTS

	Strongly disagree	Disagree	Neutral	Agree	Strongly agree
This experiment helped me find indicators that I can put on my Performance Longevity Dashboard.	○	○	○	○	○
If so, what are they?					
I noticed connections to other categories in the M3 Model.	○	○	○	○	○
If so, what were they?					
Will anything you learned in this experiment affect how you approach this aspect of your performance longevity in the future? If so, what was it?					
I would recommend this experiment to a friend or family member.	○	○	○	○	○
As a result of doing this experiment, I am more likely to continue experimenting.	○	○	○	○	○
What other experiments could you do? Write down a few examples for later reference.					
Write a brief but specific statement describing something you learned that surprised you.					

MTTR EXPERIMENTS

Experiment #1: Sleep

Quality sleep is essential for short-term performance as well as long-term health. Lots of supplements and intervention protocols get recommended, which can make it challenging to figure out what really moves the needle in the right direction.

For this experiment, you're going to use some simple tools and measure their effects on your sleep. As with most of these experiments, you'll have a variety of both indicators and tools to choose from.

Description

Run time: Fifteen days.

Using experiment indicators: The indicators for this experiment are sleep latency, phases of sleep, and restfulness during sleep, all of which can be measured with a wearable sleep tracker such as an Apple Watch or Ōura Ring. Choose one of these as your primary indicator and measure it daily. You may use more than one of the indicators if you want, but maintain a single primary indicator for the entirety of the experiment. For consistency, take measurements first thing in the morning before consuming caffeine or other stimulants and before using the tool each day.

Using experiment tools: The tools for this experiment are regular bedtime, pre-sleep ritual, self-massage, and outdoor walks. Be sure to read the instructions for each carefully.

Indicators

The indicators for this experiment require the use of a hypnogram via a wearable health-tracking device like an Apple Watch, Ōura Ring, or FitBit. For a quick review on using hypnograms to track sleep, flip back to page 206.

When you look at your hypnogram, be aware that it compresses multiple metrics into one. Here are a few to consider when looking at sleep data this way:

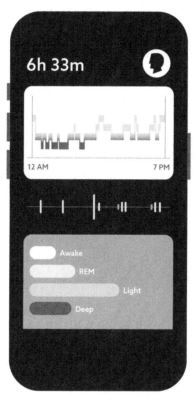

- **Latency:** Time to enter into your first sleep cycle after falling asleep.

- **Phases:** When performing your experiment, pay attention to how REM, deep, and light sleep might be differently affected by the tool you're using.

- **Restfulness:** This is a measure of how much you move around during sleep. Some sleep monitors provide an indication of restfulness along with the phases of sleep.

If you don't have access to a wearable device, take a minute each day to record the time you went to bed, the amount of time you spent in bed, and whether you felt well rested upon waking.

Tools

Regular Bedtime

Over the course of this experiment, go to bed inside the same one-hour window every night. For me, it's between 9:30 and 10:30 p.m. The timing might be different for you. That's for you to find out. Just be consistent.

Pre-Sleep Ritual

This ritual starts thirty minutes to an hour before getting into bed. For the duration of the experiment, standardize your pre-sleep behavior. Do the same things every night—read a book, hang out with loved ones, walk your dog. For the sake of this experiment, it doesn't matter what they are; just keep them the same, and do them in the same order.

Self-Massage

Use a foam roller or self-massage ball to give yourself a massage for five to ten minutes just before getting into bed. Even a tennis ball can work in a pinch.

This self-massage isn't about "getting the knots out" or making big changes. It's just to get your muscles to relax a little bit before you hop into bed. Find a few spots that need some love and attention and get in there.

Below are some easy options to start with. If you have other stretching or self-massage options you've tried before, by all means use them; just be sure you don't generate too much discomfort but instead help your body "pump the brakes" by relaxing your soft tissues.

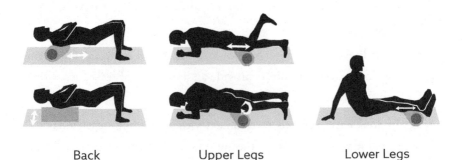

Back   Upper Legs   Lower Legs

Outdoor Walk

Walk outdoors for a minimum of fifteen minutes and a maximum of sixty minutes each day. If you can be consistent with your time, it will probably be helpful for planning purposes, but it isn't altogether necessary to walk the same number of minutes each day or to walk at the exact same time of day. Walk when it works for you.

STARTING SURVEY

Answer the following questions based on the past week of your life.

	Never	Rarely	Sometimes	Often	Always
I pay attention to how I sleep.	○	○	○	○	○
I measure my sleep with a device.	○	○	○	○	○

	Strongly disagree	Disagree	Neutral	Agree	Strongly agree
Based on these things, I've made measurable changes to my sleep habits.	○	○	○	○	○

	Never	Rarely	Sometimes	Often	Always
I have trouble getting to sleep.	○	○	○	○	○
I have trouble staying asleep.	○	○	○	○	○

I typically wake up feeling:	○ Tired	○ Fairly rested	○ Energized

	Never	Rarely	Sometimes	Often	Always
I get enough sleep.	○	○	○	○	○
I get high-quality sleep.	○	○	○	○	○

I typically sleep ____ hours per night.	○ <5	○ 5–7	○ 7–9	○ 9+

	Never	Rarely	Sometimes	Often	Always
I go outside during the day.	○	○	○	○	○
I eat close to bedtime.	○	○	○	○	○
I drink alcohol in the evening.	○	○	○	○	○
I look at electronic devices before bed.	○	○	○	○	○
I watch the news at night.	○	○	○	○	○
I toss and turn a lot in the night.	○	○	○	○	○
I snore loudly enough to disturb others.	○	○	○	○	○
I wake up grumpy.	○	○	○	○	○
If I can't have coffee, there's hell to pay.	○	○	○	○	○

I have a generally positive attitude about my sleep.	○ Strongly disagree	○ Disagree	○ Neutral	○ Agree	○ Strongly agree
Sleep is important to me.	○ Strongly disagree	○ Disagree	○ Neutral	○ Agree	○ Strongly agree

DAILY SURVEY

Take this survey in the morning each day during the experiment.

	Strongly disagree	Disagree	Neutral	Agree	Strongly agree
I went to bed on time.	○	○	○	○	○
I had trouble getting comfortable in bed.	○	○	○	○	○
I had trouble falling asleep.	○	○	○	○	○
I had trouble staying asleep.	○	○	○	○	○

MTTR EXPERIMENTS

I remember waking up ____ times.	○ 0	○ 1–3	○ 3+
I did something to try to help myself fall asleep or get back to sleep. If so, what was it?			

	Strongly disagree	Disagree	Neutral	Agree	Strongly agree
I woke up feeling energized.	○	○	○	○	○
I woke up in a good mood.	○	○	○	○	○
I feel sluggish.	○	○	○	○	○

My body feels:	○ Light	○ Heavy	○ Normal

	Strongly disagree	Disagree	Neutral	Agree	Strongly agree
I wasn't ready to be awake when I woke up.	○	○	○	○	○
I performed self-massage for ____ minutes before bed (if applicable).					
I fell asleep looking at a screen.	○	○	○	○	○
I got enough exercise yesterday.	○	○	○	○	○
I went outside yesterday.	○	○	○	○	○
I have a lot on my mind.	○	○	○	○	○
I stayed up later than I meant to.	○	○	○	○	○
I drank alcohol yesterday.	○	○	○	○	○
I had strong food cravings today.	○	○	○	○	○

I ate within ____ of bed last night.	○ 2 hours	○ 90 minutes	○ 60 minutes
I woke up to pee ____ times.	○ 0	○ 1–2	○ 3+

ENDING SURVEY AND REFLECTION QUESTIONS

Answer these questions at the end of the experiment to reflect on what you've learned. What changed? Why? What can you do next? Did something change that you didn't expect? All of these types of lessons and more as you engage!

	Never	Rarely	Sometimes	Often	Always
I pay attention to how I sleep.	O	O	O	O	O
I measure my sleep with a device.	O	O	O	O	O

	Strongly disagree	Disagree	Neutral	Agree	Strongly agree
Based on these things, I've made measurable changes to my sleep habits.	O	O	O	O	O

	Never	Rarely	Sometimes	Often	Always
I have trouble getting to sleep.	O	O	O	O	O
I have trouble staying asleep.	O	O	O	O	O

	<5	5-7	7-9	9+
I typically sleep ____ hours per night.	O	O	O	O

	Never	Rarely	Sometimes	Often	Always
I go outside during the day.	O	O	O	O	O
I eat close to bedtime.	O	O	O	O	O
I drink alcohol in the evening.	O	O	O	O	O
I look at electronic devices before bed.	O	O	O	O	O
I watch the news at night.	O	O	O	O	O
I toss and turn a lot in the night.	O	O	O	O	O

	Never	Rarely	Sometimes	Often	Always
I snore loudly enough to disturb others.	◯	◯	◯	◯	◯
I wake up grumpy.	◯	◯	◯	◯	◯
If I can't have coffee, there's hell to pay.	◯	◯	◯	◯	◯

I have a generally positive attitude about my sleep.	◯ Strongly disagree	◯ Disagree	◯ Neutral	◯ Agree	◯ Strongly agree
Sleep is important to me.	◯ Strongly disagree	◯ Disagree	◯ Neutral	◯ Agree	◯ Strongly agree

	Strongly disagree	Disagree	Neutral	Agree	Strongly agree
There have been changes in my sleep since I started this experiment.	◯	◯	◯	◯	◯
If so, what are they?					
If you share a sleeping space with others, have they reported any changes? If not, ask them. If so, what are they?					
This experiment gave me a new perspective on my sleep habits.	◯	◯	◯	◯	◯
If so, what has changed?					
This experiment has helped me make better sense of my sleep and how I can measure and change it.	◯	◯	◯	◯	◯
If so, how?					

	Strongly disagree	Disagree	Neutral	Agree	Strongly agree
I learned something important about my sleep that I'll keep using.	○	○	○	○	○
If so, briefly describe what you learned.					
This experiment helped me find indicators that I can put on my Performance Longevity Dashboard.	○	○	○	○	○
If so, what are they?					
I noticed connections to other categories in the M3 Model.	○	○	○	○	○
If so, what were they?					
Will anything you learned in this experiment affect how you approach this aspect of your performance longevity in the future? If so, what was it?					
I would recommend a sleep experiment to a friend or family member.	○	○	○	○	○
As a result of doing this experiment, I am more likely to continue experimenting.	○	○	○	○	○
What other experiments could you do? Write down a few examples for later reference.					
Write a brief but specific statement describing something you learned that surprised you.					

Experiment #2: Body Composition

A special thank you to Cheryl Zinkowski of Catalyzt Nutrition in Virginia Beach, Virginia, for her help in the design of the nutrition-based experiments.

Body composition and nutritional choices go hand in hand. The purpose of this experiment is neither to prescribe any kind of dietary or nutritional advice nor to help you achieve a specific body composition goal. If you have a precise target, you should probably seek more organized help than this workbook provides. However, the tools you'll be using for this experiment can be helpful for better attuning yourself to your perception of and interaction with the food you eat. While some of the tools may seem rudimentary, you'd be surprised to learn how many elite performers fail to use precise metrics or tools to organize themselves and, like the rest of us, often come to them only after a system failure has occurred.

Improving the nutritional quality of your food intake is a must regardless of whether you're an athlete trying to prolong performance outcomes or you just want to live a more active and fulfilling lifestyle. There are many roads to this goal, and the diet and nutrition industry has almost as much zealotry as politics and religion combined. Regardless of which style of eating appeals to you, there are some bedrock behaviors that can be helpful. Where there is wiggle room for exploration is in *how* you go about it.

If you are interested in improving your relationship with food, whether for the purpose of fat loss or muscle gain or both, the tools herein may provide reasonable starting points. The truth is, I don't know exactly what is going to work for you.

Description

Run time: Fifteen days (if using surveys only) to thirty days (if using numeric metrics like body weight or body fat percentage).

Using experiment indicators: The indicators for this experiment are DEXA scans/hydrostatic weighing, InBody scans, and body weight. Choose one of these as your primary indicator and measure once at the start of the experiment and again at the end of the fifteen to thirty days. Take measurements first thing in the morning. The body composition metrics have strict guidelines regarding consumption of food, water, and caffeine before testing. Be sure to heed the guidelines of the test facility and the professional administering the test for accurate measurements.

Using experiment tools: The tools for this experiment are macros and calories, protein intake, fiber intake, shrinking your plate, and time-restricted eating. For this experiment, you may use one tool for the entire period or try different tools for at least ten consecutive days each. If switching tools before mid-experiment, allow a two- to three-day "washout" period before starting the next one.

Note: This experiment is focused on encouraging you to be more conscious of your food choices and how they affect you. The tools listed are general recommendations that can lead to improvements in body composition. Most people are not as lean as they'd prefer to be, so the metrics and tools are primarily used to help you measure and lose body fat. If you have a different goal, please seek the help of an informed professional.

Indicators

The metrics for body composition are listed from most precise to least accurate. You will take measurements at the beginning and end of the experiment to determine changes. If you find a tool that is working for you and you want to do your retest more than thirty days after your initial test, you certainly could do so.

DEXA Scans and Hydrostatic Weighing

Dual energy X-ray absorptiometry, or DEXA, uses X-rays to determine lean mass to body fat ratio. You lie on a table for about five minutes while your body gets scanned, and then you get a report of your body composition ratio.

Hydrostatic weighing is a technique that uses volumetrics to determine your body fat to lean mass ratio by weighing you in water.

Both of these methods are generally available to the public for a fee via university exercise science labs. Depending on your location, there may be boutique health and fitness clinics that offer these services as well. A brief internet search will usually turn up any available services in your area.

InBody Scans

InBody scans use electrical current to measure skeletal muscle mass and body fat mass. Though not as accurate as DEXA or hydrostatic weighing, InBody testing can be a reliable way to keep track of trends in body composition. It is often easier to find and less expensive as well.

Body Weight

Some weight scales like the kind you can buy from your local home goods store offer a body composition metric in addition to weight. If you decide to use this option for the sake of cost effectiveness, be sure to take more frequent measurements to make up for the lack of accuracy.

If you're going to use body weight as a metric, it's important to weigh yourself first thing in the morning every day during the experiment. Your average weight at the end of each week will be your marker. The only caveat that bears mentioning here is that weighing on a daily basis makes some people feel worse psychologically and emotionally. If you know this to be true of yourself, then please use the daily survey as your primary point of reference. Women, please be cognizant of the effect your menstrual cycle may have on body weight fluctuations. Use averages!

Tools

Food Tracking

Tracking your macronutrient intake (protein, carbohydrates, and fats) and total calorie consumption can be a powerful tool for understanding and adjusting your nutrition. Instead of relying on guesswork, this tool gives you real data to help you decide where you need to make tweaks. To make this task easier, I highly recommend using a tracking app. There are many available; my personal favorite is Carbon (developed by Dr. Layne Norton), though MyFitnessPal and other free apps like it can also do the job. These apps allow you to input your body weight, body fat percentage, and activity level to estimate your daily caloric needs. The key is consistency— whichever app you choose, stick with it throughout this experiment.

Think of macro and calorie tracking like budgeting. To manage your money, you need to know how much you're earning. Tracking macros and calories is the same idea. If you don't know how much energy you're taking in or where it's coming from, it's hard to make meaningful adjustments.

For this experiment, your goal is not just to record what you eat but to make informed adjustments based on what you learn. Here's how:

- **Track before changing anything.** For the first few days, log your food intake without altering your eating habits. This gives you a baseline understanding of how you typically eat.

- **Track everything you eat.** Include snacks, condiments, and dressings, as every calorie counts. Research shows most people underestimate their intake, so logging everything, even temporarily, provides a reality check on your actual consumption.

- **Adjust as needed.** Once you have a few days of data, make small changes. If your protein intake is too low, increase it. If calories are consistently over or under your needs, adjust your portion sizes accordingly.

By using macros and calories as a tool as well as an indicator, you're actively experimenting with how adjustments in your intake affect your energy levels, performance, and overall well-being.

Nutrition is complex, but managing your diet doesn't have to be complicated. Tracking calories and macronutrient intake is just one way to take a closer look at what's going into your body and how making alterations can change how you feel and perform.

Check out the full list of recommended apps in the Resource section.

Protein Intake

Getting enough protein is a good way to start on a path toward better eating. Protein provides the highest degree of satiety of the three macronutrients. Additionally, adequate protein intake is essential for supporting the health of skeletal muscle. A general recommendation is between 0.8 and 1.2 grams of protein per kilogram of body weight, per day. So, a 150-pound (68-kilogram) person would want to consume between 54 and 82 grams each day. Ideally, most of that protein should come from sources that are lean and don't come with the baggage of a ton of saturated fat—think chicken and turkey over pork or peanut butter. Women and people over the age of sixty tend to need a little more protein to preserve healthy lean tissue, as do those who are working to build muscle. That said, it's best to do some experimenting to find out what works best for you.

As you go through this experiment, be sure to record all of your protein intake every day. Use nutrition labels when available or use apps like Carbon or Inside Tracker (both paid) or MyFitnessPal (free).

Fiber Intake

Fiber is essential for long-term health, and very few of us get enough of it. Adding fiber to your diet can be a way to get your nutrition habits on track. Fiber improves digestion, increases satiety, and provides a good environment for gut health. Good sources of fiber are whole grains, leafy greens, and cruciferous vegetables. Believe it or not, popcorn has around 15 grams of fiber per 3.5 ounces. (Just be careful not to add a bunch of junk to it and sabotage yourself.) While everyone needs sufficient fiber, both the sources and the amount consumed can affect individuals differently. Experiment with different fiber-rich foods and adjust your intake within the recommended range to see what best supports your digestion and overall health.

- **Men:** Aim for 35–45 grams of fiber per day.

- **Women:** Aim for 15–30 grams of fiber per day.

These recommendations are very broad and general. If you want recommendations that are more specific to you, work with a registered dietitian.

As you go through this experiment, be sure to record all of your fiber intake every day. Use nutrition labels or apps like Carbon, Inside Tracker, or MyFitnessPal.

Shrink Your Plate

Portion sizes in the Western world, and especially in the United States, have grown dramatically over the last generation. A simple tool to start managing nutrition and losing body fat is to use a smaller plate. Take a look at the normal dinner plate you use at home and, well, just use a smaller one. The smaller your plate, the less food you are likely to eat.

The average dinner plate is between 10 and 12 inches in diameter. Start using a dessert plate (8 to 10 inches) or an appetizer plate (6 to 8 inches) for your meals. Don't make a drastic change that you can't sustain. Choose a switch that you know you can stick to for the entire fifteen to thirty days. If you want, you can shrink your bowls and cups, too.

Remember, this isn't about building Rome in a day; it's about the net effect of all of your meals. Three meals per day for thirty days adds up to ninety meals. Even if you cut down just your dinner every day, that's thirty opportunities to reduce your calorie intake.

Time-Restricted Eating (TRE)

Time-restricted eating, sometimes referred to as intermittent fasting, is the purposeful limitation of eating to a specific block of time each day. During this "feeding window," there are no specific restrictions on what you eat. The feeding window is generally between six and twelve hours long, and for the rest of the twenty-four-hour period, you consume no food or drinks other than water and maybe some tea.

Which span of time you choose to designate as your feeding window will depend on what works best for your life. This will undoubtedly require some trial and error. A good place to start is taking into consideration energy demands for work and exercise as well as important social engagements like dinner with your family. What's most important is to find a schedule that allows for consistency and doesn't add unnecessary stress to your life.

Note: While all of the tools presented here are based on valid scientific consensus, be sure to check with your healthcare provider beforehand if you are managing any health conditions or have doubts about what is right for you.

STARTING SURVEY

Answer the following questions based on the past week of your life.

I read food labels.	○ Never	○ When I already think the food is healthy	○ Sometimes	○ Always

I have a good sense of what food labels mean.	○ Strongly disagree	○ Disagree	○ Neutral	○ Agree	○ Strongly agree

I record my food intake.	○ Never	○ Only when I feel like my health has gotten away from me	
	○ Often	○ Sometimes	○ Always

It's most important that my food:	○ Is healthy	○ Tastes good	○ Smells good

I want my food to be:	○ Cheap	○ Expensive	○ Good value for the price

I eat the same things every day.	○ Strongly disagree	○ Disagree	○ Neutral	○ Agree	○ Strongly agree

The food I eat is:	○ Low in calories	○ High in calories	○ I don't know

My food *(select all that apply)*:	⭘ Helps me relax	⭘ Cheers me up	⭘ Makes me feel good
	⭘ Helps me cope with stress		⭘ Rewards me for hard work

My food *(select all that apply)*:	⭘ Is nutritious	⭘ Is high in protein
	⭘ Is high in fiber	⭘ Contains a lot of vitamins and minerals

I have watery stool.	⭘ Strongly disagree	⭘ Disagree	⭘ Neutral	⭘ Agree	⭘ Strongly agree

My stool floats.	⭘ Strongly disagree	⭘ Disagree	⭘ Neutral	⭘ Agree	⭘ Strongly agree

My stool sinks.	⭘ Strongly disagree	⭘ Disagree	⭘ Neutral	⭘ Agree	⭘ Strongly agree

I pass feces:	⭘ Once a week	⭘ Every 3 days	⭘ Less than once per day
	⭘ Once per day	⭘ 2–3x per day	⭘ 4+x per day

	Strongly disagree	Disagree	Neutral	Agree	Strongly agree
I pass gas.	⭘	⭘	⭘	⭘	⭘
I have sudden and unexpected bowel movements.	⭘	⭘	⭘	⭘	⭘
When I defecate, it takes a long time.	⭘	⭘	⭘	⭘	⭘
When I defecate, it is effortful.	⭘	⭘	⭘	⭘	⭘
When I defecate, it is painful.	⭘	⭘	⭘	⭘	⭘

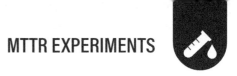

DAILY SURVEY

Take this survey at the end of each day during the experiment.

	Strongly disagree	Disagree	Neutral	Agree	Strongly agree
I did the experiment as written today.	○	○	○	○	○
I ate the same thing as yesterday.	○	○	○	○	○
(Skip if not using body weight as a metric) I weighed myself.	○	○	○	○	○
I had a hard time sticking to the plan.	○	○	○	○	○
I ate poorly.	○	○	○	○	○
I got enough sleep last night.	○	○	○	○	○
I've been feeling stressed.	○	○	○	○	○
I have a lot going on, so I couldn't eat right.	○	○	○	○	○
I exercised.	○	○	○	○	○
I was more active than usual.	○	○	○	○	○
I felt bad about something I ate.	○	○	○	○	○
I made a conscious choice to eat something less nutritious.	○	○	○	○	○
I ate at a social event or celebration.	○	○	○	○	○
What did you get right?					
How can you build on that success?					

What could have gone better?	
What could nothing be done about?	
What leading indicators might there be that will help you stay on track?	

ENDING SURVEY AND REFLECTION QUESTIONS

Answer these questions after completing the experiment to reflect on what you've learned. What changed? Why? What can you do next? Did something change that you didn't expect? All of these types of lessons and more as you engage!

I read food labels.				
	○ Never	○ When I already think the food is healthy	○ Sometimes	○ Always

I have a good sense of what food labels mean.				
	○ Strongly disagree	○ Disagree	○ Neutral	○ Agree	○ Strongly agree

I record my food intake:		
	○ Never	○ Only when I feel like my health has gotten away from me
	○ Often	○ Sometimes	○ Always

It's most important that my food:			
	○ Is healthy	○ Tastes good	○ Smells good

I want my food to be:			
	○ Cheap	○ Expensive	○ Good value for the price

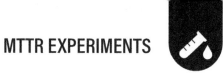

I eat the same things every day.	◯ Strongly disagree	◯ Disagree	◯ Neutral	◯ Agree	◯ Strongly agree

The food I eat is:	◯ Low in calories		◯ High in calories		◯ I don't know

My food (select all that apply):	◯ Helps me relax		◯ Cheers me up		◯ Makes me feel good
		◯ Helps me cope with stress			◯ Rewards me for hard work

I performed the experiment as written _____ days per week.	◯ 1–3	◯ 3–5	◯ 6–7

	Strongly disagree	Disagree	Neutral	Agree	Strongly agree
This experiment helped me make better sense of my relationship with food.	◯	◯	◯	◯	◯
I learned something important about my food choices and how they affect me.	◯	◯	◯	◯	◯
(Skip if not your metric) I saw a positive change in my body composition.	◯	◯	◯	◯	◯
The experiment helped me find indicators that I can put on my Performance Longevity Dashboard.	◯	◯	◯	◯	◯
If so, what are they?					
I noticed connections to other categories in the M3 Model.	◯	◯	◯	◯	◯
If so, what were they?					

Will anything you learned in this experiment affect how you approach this aspect of your performance longevity in the future? If so, what was it?					
	Strongly disagree	Disagree	Neutral	Agree	Strongly agree
I would recommend this experiment to a friend or family member.	○	○	○	○	○
As a result of doing this experiment, I am more likely to continue experimenting.	○	○	○	○	○
What other experiments could you do? Write down a few examples for later reference.					
Write a brief but specific statement describing something you learned that surprised you.					

Experiment #3: Aerobic Health

The efficient and effective delivery of oxygen to the brain and body is an essential part of performance longevity. If you read that out loud, it sounds as obvious as sunshine, but very few people, including both athletes and regular folks just trying to be healthy, have the first clue about how well their bodies are delivering oxygen. You could make some presumptions, but as always, it's better to have some metrics that you can rely on.

Please know that, like the rest of the options for both tools and indicators put forth in this book, the purpose here is to attune yourself to the reality of what is happening in your brain and body. Once you develop a relationship with an indicator or tool that makes sense to you, it's up to you to continue to pursue those aspects to their end point of benefit. For example, because a wide range of aerobic fitness levels can be represented at the start of this experiment, a wide variety of outcomes are possible. Don't forget that the point is to find an indicator, use a tool that you think will alter your measurements, and then revisit your hypothesis to determine what adjustments you can make in your approach to solving that problem or achieving that goal.

A note for those of you who fancy yourselves fit or well-conditioned: You're probably not as efficient as you could be. I have worked with many elite athletes who excelled in their sport but were not at all efficient at using oxygen. They had no idea that this was the case until they were tested. If you are fit enough that the metrics listed below are insufficient, consider going to a nearby university's exercise physiology department and getting your VO2 max tested. It can be an eye-opening process.

If you do not desire or need that level of precision, there are some substitutes that will do the job. These metrics are probably good enough if you're not already engaged in regular and purposeful aerobic conditioning work.

Description

Run time: Thirty days. The structure is based on your current level of aerobic activity.

Using experiment indicators: The indicators for this experiment are VO2 max, fixed-time test, fixed-distance test, heart rate recovery, and resting heart rate. Select one of these as your primary indicator and measure it daily at the same time of day. You may track additional indicators, but maintain consistency with one primary metric throughout the experiment. For accuracy, take measurements first thing in the morning before consuming caffeine or other stimulants and before using your chosen tool.

Using experiment tools: The tools for this experiment are walking and HIIT/MICT. The experiment is divided into two categories, and how you use the tool(s) will depend on which category you fall into:

- *Active:* If you already engage in purposeful aerobic exercise at least two days per week and have been for at least a year, select one tool and use it consistently for the full thirty-day period. Train three to five days per week, totaling between twelve and twenty sessions.

Schedule your exercise days in a way that fits your routine.

- *Inactive:* If you are not currently engaged in regular aerobic activity, you may switch tools each week if desired. Use your chosen tool two to four days per week, maintaining consistency within each week.

Regardless of category, maintain consistency in timing and effort.

Indicators

VO2 Max

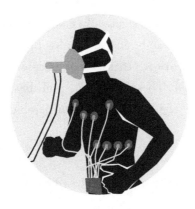

VO2 max is the maximum volume of oxygen your body can use. It is measured in milliliters per kilogram per minute (ml/kg/min). Your VO2 max is determined through the use of an exercise test that you perform on a piece of exercise equipment with calibrated work rates, like a treadmill or specialized stationary bike, while wearing a mask that measures oxygen and carbon dioxide exchange to determine how effectively your body is using energy. The tester uses data from the gas exchange, work rate, heart rate, and body weight to determine your energy expenditure and deliver a score that can be compared to the scores of others in your age group.

VO2 max tests, while accurate, can be difficult to access for many people. If you have a college or university nearby, you may be able to make an appointment in their exercise physiology lab to get tested. If you're not ready to go there quite yet, check out some of the proxy aerobic tests that follow.

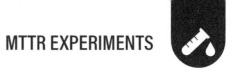

Fixed-Time Test

A fixed-time test measures the maximum distance covered in a set amount of time. The Cooper Test is an example of this kind of metric. In the Cooper Test, you cover as much distance as you can in twelve minutes. Ideally, such a test is done on a standard track—i.e., 400-meter loops—but you could do a fixed-time test anywhere the terrain is constant and you can measure the distance you traveled. My home city of Virginia Beach, Virginia, has an oceanfront boardwalk that is 3 miles long and as such serves as a great way for locals to measure their fitness. If you wanted to do a fixed-time test, you could set a timer and see how far down the boardwalk you could walk, jog, run, or some mixture thereof. Lots of wearables and smartphone apps have ways to determine distance covered.

Even more simply, you could set a timer for twelve minutes and see how many flights of stairs you could climb in that time. Be creative! Just make sure that whatever test you use as your marker, you compare it only to itself. Make note of the test conditions, including both things that could affect your state of body and mind (higher than normal stress or lack of sleep, for example) as well as things in the environment that might affect the outcome (such as windy weather or a rain-slicked testing surface).

Fixed-Distance Test

Using fixed distance is very similar to fixed time, but instead of having a countdown clock and covering as much distance as possible, you use a timer to determine how long it takes you to cover a set distance. Think back to the mile run from high school PE class, for example. That's what I mean.

If you were here in Virginia Beach, you could walk, jog, or run the 3-mile boardwalk and time your effort year over year as a personal measure of aerobic capacity. While you don't necessarily need to cover 3 miles, it is important to stretch your effort from twelve to twenty-plus minutes to get a decent read on your aerobic system.

If you use this metric as your dashboard indicator for aerobic health, the key is consistency—pick a set distance, try to cover it as quickly as possible, and use that metric for comparison over time. Just as with fixed-time tests, you could also apply this principle to other efforts, such as stair climbs. Instead of seeing how many flights you can complete in a fixed period, you could time how long it takes you to climb a set number of flights. This ensures you're measuring your progress in a way that aligns with your environment and goals.

2-Kilometer Walk Test

The 2-kilometer (1.24-mile) walk is a widely accepted fixed-distance test for fitness if you find yourself unable to run. You simply walk 2 kilometers as fast as you can and record your time and your heart rate (HR) at the end. After a period of consistent aerobic exercise, you retest to compare your time and ending heart rate.

If you want to be a bit more of an Engineer about it, you can use these equations to determine a proxy VO2 max:

- **Men:** VO2 max (ml/min/kg) = $184.9 - (4.65 \times \text{walk time}) - (0.22 \times \text{HR}) - (0.26 \times \text{age}) - (1.05 \times \text{BMI})$

- **Women:** VO2 max (ml/min/kg) = $116.2 - (2.98 \times \text{walk time}) - (0.11 \times \text{HR}) - (0.14 \times \text{age}) - (0.39 \times \text{BMI})$

Source: EuroFit Walk Test

Other examples of accessible fixed-time tests include the Rockport Test and the 1-Mile Walk Test. To do many of these types of tests, all that's required is a heart rate monitor and a timer. Both are embedded in many modern wearable devices, but they are also available at low cost at most sporting goods stores.

As a heads-up, if you've never done any kind of aerobic test before, they're hard. If you lollygag through it and don't produce real effort—and only *you* can know if you are—not only will the test not reflect your ability, but any intervention based on that metric will be rendered far less potent.

You may have noticed that I didn't provide a good/better/best for the fixed-time and fixed-distance tests. First, I have no idea who you are or what your specific needs might be. If you want some general guidelines, check out the Cooper Institute. Additionally, unless you compete as an endurance athlete, the most important thing is to stay tuned in to your metrics over time and do your best to improve them or at least not let them atrophy.

Most of these metrics can be scaled to fit any level of experience. There are some obvious exceptions: For example, if you have been running for exercise three days per week for years, a walk test isn't going to provide enough of a challenge. With that said, some of the other metrics could provide insight, especially when combined with the add-on metrics below.

The following can be used, regardless of skill or fitness level, as either add-ons or standalone metrics.

Heart Rate Recovery

Heart rate recovery (HRR) is the beats-per-minute decrease in your heart rate one, two, and three minutes after stopping exercise, with the one-minute marker being the most commonly used metric. To measure HRR, you use a heart rate monitor chest strap or one that is embedded in a wearable device.

Immediately after stopping exercise, measure your heart rate at its peak. Then, after one minute, measure your heart rate again, and subtract that number from your peak heart rate to get your HRR. You can repeat this process at the two- and three-minute marks (post-exercise) as well. Be sure to subtract those numbers from your peak heart rate, not from the one- and two-minute measurements.

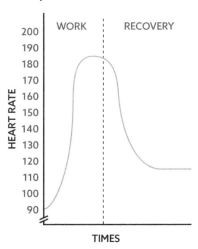

Resting Heart Rate

Your resting heart rate is the lowest heart rate you experience in the course of a day. Usually, your heart rate is lowest during sleep. Many wearable devices will calculate this number for you. If you don't have access to a wearable device, simply take your pulse in the morning immediately upon waking. If you use a digital blood pressure monitor or pulse oximeter for any reason, those devices can measure heart rate as well. Please realize that digital heart rate monitors can vary significantly, so whichever one you are using to determine your resting heart rate, it is important to consistently use *that device* for that purpose.

Resting heart rate does not strongly correlate to VO2 max in particular, but it is a reliable leading indicator for cardiovascular health. Most people have a resting heart rate between 60 and 100 bpm, with lots of reasons as to why. As a general rule, an RHR below 60 bpm is desirable for athletes and active people, but if you have a low resting heart rate and a history of a circulatory disorder, it may be a reason to seek out medical help to be sure everything is functioning well.

None of the above proxies is as precise as a legitimate VO2 max test. However, they can serve as good places to start accruing data about how well your body is using energy, especially if you combine an exercise test with heart rate recovery and resting heart rate data. Those three together will probably provide a "good enough" set of indicators for aerobic health for the vast majority of people trying to stay healthy. If you're a true Engineer type, pony up the cash for a VO2 max test.

Tools

Any and all tools that help improve the way the body uses oxygen involve exercise. You have to get moving and ask for adaptation. Unfortunately, these adaptations can be uncomfortable, especially if you haven't been routinely challenging your body in productive ways. Having said that, the rewards of a healthy aerobic system are manifold and will pay huge dividends in both quality and quantity of performance longevity.

Walking

Walking is a simple and accessible way to start improving aerobic health. If you are already very fit, improvements in VO2 max from walking may be marginal at best, but for mere mortals looking to stay generally healthy, walking is a great starting point.

While there is no magic number for steps, there does seem to be an inverse relationship between steps taken and health markers. The general recommendation is 8,000 to 10,000 steps per day, totaling around 4 to 5 miles. If you're starting from zero, try to get in 5,000 steps a day a few days a week and see what happens, and then build up from there.

Note: If you're already relatively fit, you can spice your walking up by carrying a loaded backpack or rucksack.

High-Intensity Interval Training (HIIT) and Moderate-Intensity Continuous Training (MICT)

High-intensity interval training and moderate-intensity continuous training are two modes of exercise that can yield improvements in aerobic performance. While the exact effects of each depend on a multitude of factors, including how fit you are to begin with, your age, and your gender, there are some general guidelines that seem to work for the vast majority of people.

High-intensity interval training is characterized by repeated bouts of high-effort work lasting thirty seconds or less with a short rest period of up to thirty seconds in between. Nearly any activity works here, presuming it is safe and allows for consistency in high effort—for example, using a stationary bike or other piece of cardio equipment, running, jogging, or climbing stairs. One of the primary benefits of HIIT is that it takes far less time than steady-state cardiovascular exercise, and the results tend to come pretty fast. This logistical advantage is a big deal for those of us who can't sit on a stationary bike for three hours a week.

While HIIT has been shown to drastically improve VO2 max in short order, it is less effective at producing aerobic change than moderate-intensity continuous training. MICT involves maintaining a steady pace of work over a longer period, usually fifteen to twenty minutes, although some experts recommend upward of 180 minutes per week. A great place to start is Zone 2 training, which is often defined as working at conversational pace—meaning if you're teetering on the edge of being able to hold a conversation while you're working, you're in the sweet spot. Usually, this state is measured through heart rate or rate of perceived exertion (how hard you feel you're working). Though it's not as convenient as HIIT, MICT yields much better aerobic results.

Longevity expert Dr. Peter Attia has volumes of information on this topic in his book *Outlive* as well as his many podcasts on the subject, which are available on YouTube for free. I highly recommend seeking out these resources if you want to do a deep dive.

Playtime

Another way to get in some aerobic work is through play. Join a kickball league (not for the beer), take up golf, or sign up for a jiu-jitsu class. All of these activities are centered around community and include elements of fun, taking your mind off the fact that you're doing aerobic exercise.

Even if you're more attracted to the idea of getting in better aerobic shape through a social avenue, it can be helpful to use a metric for a period of time to see if and how that activity is affecting you. We all need to calibrate our perception!

STARTING SURVEY

Answer the following questions based on the past week of your life.

Aerobic health is an important part of my current health and performance program.	○ Strongly disagree	○ Disagree	○ Neutral	○ Agree	○ Strongly agree

I perform purposeful aerobic exercise _____ days per week.	○ 0	○ 1–2	○ 3	○ 4+

	Strongly disagree	Disagree	Neutral	Agree	Strongly agree
I experience shortness of breath if I have to exert myself.	○	○	○	○	○
Once my heart rate goes up, it takes a long time to come down.	○	○	○	○	○
I get fatigued by everyday activities.	○	○	○	○	○

My aerobic fitness is:	○ Very poor	○ Poor	○ Acceptable	○ Good	○ Excellent
How do you know?					

I purposefully seek out opportunities to make myself work aerobically (for example, I park far away, take the stairs instead of the elevator, ride a bike to dinner, etc.).	○ Strongly disagree	○ Disagree	○ Neutral	○ Agree	○ Strongly agree

I take part in leisure activities that have an element of aerobic activity (play pickleball, Frisbee, golf, walk my dog).	○ Strongly disagree	○ Disagree	○ Neutral	○ Agree	○ Strongly agree
If so, what are they?	_____ _____				

I do these activities _____ days per week.	○ 0	○ 1–2	○ 3	○ 4+

I get pretty bad muscle cramps when I exercise.	○ Strongly disagree	○ Disagree	○ Neutral	○ Agree	○ Strongly agree

DAILY SURVEY

Take this survey at the end of each day during the experiment.

	Strongly disagree	Disagree	Neutral	Agree	Strongly agree
I did some aerobic work today.	○	○	○	○	○
I got muscle cramps.	○	○	○	○	○
I didn't want to exercise but did anyway.	○	○	○	○	○

My sleep last night was:	○ Very poor	○ Poor	○ Acceptable	○ Good	○ Excellent

My energy level today was:	○ Very poor	○ Poor	○ Acceptable	○ Good	○ Excellent

I had a stressful day yesterday.	○ Strongly disagree	○ Disagree	○ Neutral	○ Agree	○ Strongly agree

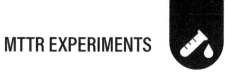

I ate ___ meal(s) with fruits and vegetables today.	○ 0	○ 1	○ 2	○ 3+	
I drank _____ 8-ounce glasses of water today.	○ 0	○ 1–3	○ 3–5	○ 5–8	○ 9+

ENDING SURVEY AND REFLECTION QUESTIONS

Answer these questions after completing the experiment to reflect on what you've learned. What changed? Why? What can you do next? Did something change that you didn't expect? All of these types of lessons and more as you engage!

Aerobic health is an important part of my current health and performance program.	○ Strongly disagree	○ Disagree	○ Neutral	○ Agree	○ Strongly agree

I perform purposeful aerobic exercise _____ days per week.	○ 0	○ 1–2	○ 3	○ 4+

	Strongly disagree	Disagree	Neutral	Agree	Strongly agree
I experience shortness of breath if I have to exert myself.	○	○	○	○	○
Once my heart rate goes up, it takes a long time to come down.	○	○	○	○	○
I get fatigued by everyday activities.	○	○	○	○	○

My aerobic fitness is:	○ Very poor	○ Poor	○ Acceptable	○ Good	○ Excellent
How do you know?					

I purposefully seek out opportunities to make myself work aerobically (for example, I park far away, take the stairs instead of the elevator, ride a bike to dinner, etc.).	◯ Strongly disagree	◯ Disagree	◯ Neutral	◯ Agree	◯ Strongly agree

I take part in leisure activities that have an element of aerobic activity (play pickleball, Frisbee, golf, walk my dog, etc.).	◯ Strongly disagree	◯ Disagree	◯ Neutral	◯ Agree	◯ Strongly agree
If so, what are they?	_____ _____				

I do these activities _____ days per week.	◯ 0	◯ 1-2	◯ 3	◯ 4+

	Strongly disagree	Disagree	Neutral	Agree	Strongly agree
I get pretty bad muscle cramps when I exercise.	◯	◯	◯	◯	◯
This experiment gave me a new perspective on my exercise habits.	◯	◯	◯	◯	◯
This experiment helped me make better sense of my aerobic health and how I can measure and change it.	◯	◯	◯	◯	◯
If so, briefly describe what you learned.	_____ _____				
I learned something important about my aerobic health that I'll keep using.	◯	◯	◯	◯	◯
If so, briefly describe what you learned.	_____ _____				

	Strongly disagree	Disagree	Neutral	Agree	Strongly agree
This experiment helped me find indicators that I can put on my Performance Longevity Dashboard.	○	○	○	○	○
If so, what were they?					
I noticed connections to other categories in the M3 Model.	○	○	○	○	○
If so, what were they?					
Will anything you learned in this experiment affect how you approach this aspect of your performance longevity in the future?	○	○	○	○	○
If so, what was it?					
I would recommend this experiment to a friend or family member.	○	○	○	○	○
As a result of doing this experiment, I am more likely to continue experimenting.	○	○	○	○	○
What other experiments could you do? Write down a few examples for later reference.					
Write a brief but specific statement describing something you learned that surprised you.					

RESOURCES

CHAPTER 1

Eurella Vest, Megan Armstrong, Vanessa A. Olbrecht, Rajan K. Thakkar, Renata B. Fabia, Jonathan I. Groner, Dana Noffsinger, Nguyen K. Tram, and Henry Xiang, "Association of Pre-Procedural Anxiety with Procedure-Related Pain During Outpatient Pediatric Burn Care: A Pilot Study," *Journal of Burn Care & Research: Official Publication of the American Burn Association* 44, no. 3 (2022): 610–617.

CHAPTER 2

Occupational Safety and Health Administration (OSHA), *Using Leading Indicators to Improve Safety and Health Outcomes,* OSHA Publication 3970, Washington, D.C.: U.S. Department of Labor, 2019.

Bryan Shipley, "Understanding Leading and Lagging Indicators," *InFocus: Research and Industry News from Arnerich Massena,* January 2019.

WorkForce Central, "Trend Analysis: Module 2," October 2017.

Michael F. Stumborg, Timothy D. Blasius, Steven J. Full, and Christine A. Hughes, "Goodhart's Law: Recognizing and Mitigating Manipulation of Measures in Analysis," Center for Naval Analyses (CNA), September 2022.

ModelThinkers, "Goodhart's Law," https://modelthinkers.com/mental-model/goodharts-law, accessed April 28, 2025.

Tableau, "What Is a Dashboard?" https://www.tableau.com/dashboard/what-is-dashboard, accessed April 25, 2025.

USA Pickleball, "Pickleball Elbow: Don't Just Ice and Rest! Fix the Mechanics!" https://usapickleball.org/member-news/pickleball-elbow-dont-just-ice-and-rest-fix-the-mechanics/, August 16, 2018.

CHAPTER 3

White House Council of Economic Advisers, "Issue Brief: Supply Chain Resilience," November 30, 2023.

Judit Monostori, "Supply Chains' Robustness: Challenges and Opportunities," *Procedia CIRP* 67 (2018): 110–115.

Marcus J. Sharman, Andrew G. Cresswell, and Stephan Riek, "Proprioceptive Neuromuscular Facilitation Stretching: Mechanisms and Clinical Implications," *Sports Medicine* 36, no. 11 (2006): 929–939.

CHAPTER 4

Jaak Panskepp, *Affective Neuroscience: The Foundations of Human and Animal Emotions* (Cambridge: Oxford University Press, September 30, 2004).

Mary Helen Immordino-Yang, *Emotions, Learning, and the Brain: Exploring the Educational Implications of Affective Neuroscience* (New York: W. W. Norton & Company, 2015).

Kay M. Tye, "Neural Circuit Motifs in Valence Processing," *Neuron* 100, no. 2 (2018): 436–452.

Adele Diamond, "Executive Functions," *Annual Review of Psychology* 64 (2013): 135–168.

Abdullah A. Alarfaj, Abdulrahman Khalid Aldrweesh, Alghaydaa Fouad Aldoughan, Sumaia Mohammed Alarfaj, Fatimah Khalid Alabdulqader, and Khalid A. Alyahya, "Olfactory Dysfunction Following COVID-19 and the Potential Benefits of Olfactory Training," *Journal of Clinical Medicine* 12, no. 14 (2023): 4761.

Li-Jung Lin and Kuan-yi Li, "Comparing the Effects of Olfactory-Based Sensory Stimulation and Board Game Training on Cognition, Emotion, and Blood Biomarkers Among Individuals with Dementia: A Pilot Randomized Controlled Trial," *Frontiers in Psychology* 13 (2022): 1003325.

Bruce S. McEwen and John C. Wingfield, "The Concept of Allostasis in Biology and Biomedicine," *Hormones and Behavior* 43, no. 1 (2003): 2–15.

Mary Helen Immordino-Yang, Joanna A. Christodoulou, and Vanessa Singh, "Rest Is Not Idleness: Implications of the Brain's Default Mode for Human Development and Education," *Perspectives on Psychological Science* 7, no. 4 (2012): 352–364.

Gernot Ernst, "Heart-Rate Variability—More Than Heart Beats?" *Frontiers in Public Health* 5 (2017): 240.

Fred Shaffer and J. P. Ginsberg, "An Overview of Heart Rate Variability Metrics and Norms," *Frontiers in Public Health* 5 (2017): 258.

Jody Ann Coore, "Emotional and Attentional Regulation: Impact of Trauma and Journal Writing?" *The Nebraska Educator,* May 2022.

Joshua M. Smyth, Jillian A. Johnson, Brandon J. Auer, Erik Lehman, Giampaolo Talamo, and Christopher N. Sciamanna, "Online Positive Affect Journaling in the Improvement of Mental Distress and Well-Being in General Medical Patients With Elevated Anxiety Symptoms: A Preliminary Randomized Controlled Trial," *JMIR Mental Health* 5, no. 4 (2018): e11290.

P. Ullrich and S. Lutgendorf, "Journaling About Stressful Events: Effects of Cognitive Processing and Emotional Expression," *Annals of Behavioral Medicine* 24 (2002): 244–250.

Dexing Zhang, Eric K. P. Lee, Eva C. W. Mak, C. Y. Ho, and Samuel Y. S. Wong, "Mindfulness-Based Interventions: An Overall Review," *British Medical Bulletin* 138, no. 1 (2021): 41–57.

Larissa Bartlett, Angela J. Martin, A. Neil, K. Memish, P. Otáhal, M. Kilpatrick, and Kristy Sanderson, "A Systematic Review and Meta-Analysis of Workplace Mindfulness Training Randomized Controlled Trials," *Journal of Occupational Health Psychology* 24, no. 1 (2019): 108–126.

Denise C. Park, Jennifer Lodi-Smith, L. Drew, Sara Haber, Andrew Hebrank, Gérard N. Bischof, and Whitley Aamodt, "The Impact of Sustained Engagement on Cognitive Function in Older Adults," *Psychological Science* 25, no. 1 (2014): 103–112.

Andrew W. Bailey and Hyoung-Kil Kang, "Walking and Sitting Outdoors: Which Is Better for Cognitive Performance and Mental States?" *International Journal of Environmental Research and Public Health* 19, no. 24 (2022): 16638.

CHAPTER 5

Jon H. Kaas, "The Evolution of the Complex Sensory and Motor Systems of the Human Brain," *Brain Research Bulletin* 75, no. 2–4 (2007): 384–390.

National Institute of Neurological Disorders and Stroke (NINDS), "Pain," https://www.ninds.nih.gov/health-information/disorders/pain accessed April 25, 2025.

Stuart McMillan, "The ALTIS Kinogram Method," *SimpliFaster,* https://simplifaster.com/articles/altis-kinogram-method/, accessed April 25, 2025.

CHAPTER 6

Anna B. Fishbein, Kristen L. Knutson, and Phyllis C. Zee, "Circadian Disruption and Human Health," *Journal of Clinical Investigation* 131, no. 19 (2021): e148286.

C. Tabor and K. R. Peeler, "Sleep Is a Human Right, and Its Deprivation Is Torture," *AMA Journal of Ethics* 26, no. 10 (2024): E784–794.

Diane B. Boivin, Philippe Boudreau, and Anastasi Kosmadopoulos, "Disturbance of the Circadian System in Shift Work and Its Health Impact," *Journal of Biological Rhythms* 37, no. 1 (2021): 3–28.

Marco Fabbri, Alessia Beracci, Monica Martoni, Debora Meneo, Lorenzo Tonetti, and Vincenzo Natale, "Measuring Subjective Sleep Quality: A Review," *International Journal of Environmental Research and Public Health* 18, no. 3 (2021): 1082.

Ari Shechter, Elijah Wookhyn Kim, Marie-Pierre St-Onge, and Andrew J. Westwood, "Blocking Nocturnal Blue Light for Insomnia: A Randomized Controlled Trial," *Journal of Psychiatric Research* 96 (2018): 196–202.

Landon Hester, Deanna H. Dang, Christopher J Barker, Michael Heath, Sidra Mesiya, Tekenari Tienabeso, and Kevin Watson, "Evening Wear of Blue-Blocking Glasses for Sleep and Mood Disorders: A Systematic Review," *Chronobiology International* 38 (2021): 1375–1383.

Lisa A. Ostrin, "Ocular and Systemic Melatonin and the Influence of Light Exposure," *Clinical and Experimental Optometry* 102, no. 2 (2019): 99–108.

Leena Tähkämö, T. Partonen, and A. Pesonen, "Systematic Review of Light Exposure Impact on Human Circadian Rhythm," *Chronobiology International* 36 (2018): 151–170.

Jeremy A. Bigalke, Ian M. Greenlund, Jennifer R. Nicevski, and Jason R. Carter, "Effect of Evening Blue Light Blocking Glasses on Subjective and Objective Sleep in Healthy Adults: A Randomized Control Trial," *Sleep Health* 7, no. 4 (2021): 485–490.

L. Lan, K. Tsuzuki, Y. F. Liu, and Z. W. Lian, "Thermal Environment and Sleep Quality: A Review," *Energy & Buildings* 149 (2017): 101–113.

Daisy Duan, Chenjuan Gu, Vsevolod Polotsky, Jonathan C. Jun, and Luu V. Pham, "Effects of Dinner Timing on Sleep Stage Distribution and EEG Power Spectrum in Healthy Volunteers," *Nature and Science of Sleep* 13 (2021): 601–612.

Chenjuan Gu, Nga Brereton, Amy Schweitzer, Matthew Cotter, Daisy Duan, Elisabet Børsheim, Robert R. Wolfe, Luu V. Pham, Vsevolod Polotsky, and Jonathan C. Jun, "Metabolic Effects of Late Dinner in Healthy Volunteers—A Randomized Crossover Clinical Trial," *Journal of Clinical Endocrinology and Metabolism* 105, no. 8 (2020): 2789–2802.

Nikola Chung, Yu Sun Bin, Peter A. Cistulli, and Chin Moi Chow, "Does the Proximity of Meals to Bedtime Influence the Sleep of Young Adults? A Cross-Sectional Survey of University Students," *International Journal of Environmental Research and Public Health* 17, no. 8 (2020): 2677.

Filipa Almeida, Daniel R. Marques, and Ana A. Gomes, "A Preliminary Study on the Association Between Social Media at night and Sleep Quality: The Relevance of FOMO, Cognitive Pre-Sleep Arousal, and Maladaptive Cognitive Emotion Regulation," *Scandinavian Journal of Psychology* 64, no. 2 (2023): 123–132.

Jean-Phillippe Chaput, Caroline Dutil, Ryan Featherstone, Robert Ross, Lora Giangregorio, Travis J. Saunders, Ian Janssen, Veronica J. Poitras, Michelle E. Kho, Amanda Ross-White, Sarah Zankar, and Julie Carrier, "Sleep Timing, Sleep Consistency, and Health in Adults: A Systematic Review," *Applied Physiology, Nutrition, and Metabolism (Physiologie Appliquee, Nutrition et Metabolisme)* 45, no. 10 (Suppl. 2) (2020): S232–S247.

Kristy L. Larsen and Sara Jordan, "Factors Associated with Consistent Bedtime Routines and Good Sleep Outcomes," *Children's Health Care* 51, no. 2 (2021): 139–162.

Elizabeth Capezuti, Kevin Pain, Evelyn Alamag, XinQing Chen, Valicia Philibert, and Ana C. Krieger, "Systematic Review: Auditory Stimulation and Sleep," *Journal of Clinical Sleep Medicine: Official Publication of the American Academy of Sleep Medicine* 18, no. 6 (2021): 1697–1709.

Mathias Basner and Sarah McGuire, "WHO Environmental Noise Guidelines for the European Region: A Systematic Review on Environmental Noise and Effects on Sleep," *International Journal of Environmental Research and Public Health* 15, no. 3 (2018): 519.

Mathias Basner, Uwe Müller, and Eva-Maria Elmenhorst, "Single and Combined Effects of Air, Road, and Rail Traffic Noise on Sleep and Recuperation," *Sleep* 34, no. 1 (2011): 11–23.

Nantawachara Jirakittayakorn and Yodchanan Wongsawat, "A Novel Insight of Effects of a 3-Hz Binaural Beat on Sleep Stages During Sleep," *Frontiers in Human Neuroscience* 12 (2018): 387.

Melisa A. Gantt, "Study Protocol to Support the Development of an All-Night Binaural Beat Frequency Audio Program to Entrain Sleep," *Frontiers in Neurology* 14 (2023): 1024726.

Suhyeon Kim, Kyungae Jo, Ki-Bae Hong, Sung He Han, and Hyung Joo Suh, "GABA and L-Theanine Mixture Decreases Sleep Latency and Improves NREM Sleep," *Pharmaceutical Biology* 57, no. 1 (2019): 65–73.

Stella Alice Oliveira Paredes Moreira, Wandemberg Farias de Albuquerque Neto, Gabriela Palitot Lourenço, Carla Liandra Ferreira da Costa, Sávio Lucas Lacerda de Araújo, and D. Barros, "Anxiolytic Effects of Oral Administration of L-Theanine: A Revision," *Proceedings of MOL2NET 2018, International Conference on Multidisciplinary Sciences,* 4th Edition.

Oliviero Bruni, Luigi Ferini-Strambi, Elena Giacomoni, and Paolo Pellegrino, "Herbal Remedies and Their Possible Effect on the GABAergic System and Sleep," *Nutrients* 13, no. 2 (2021): 530.

Mounir Chennaoui, Pierrick Arnal, Fabien Sauvet, and Damien Léger, "Sleep and Exercise: A Reciprocal Issue?" *Sleep Medicine Reviews* 20 (2015): 59–72.

Sohrab Amiri, Jafar Hasani, and Mojtaba Satkin, "Effect of Exercise Training on Improving Sleep Disturbances: A Systematic Review and Meta-Analysis of Randomized Control Trials," *Sleep Medicine* 84 (2021): 205–218.

Perry Nicassio and Richard Bootzin, "A Comparison of Progressive Relaxation and Autogenic Training as Treatments for Insomnia," *Journal of Abnormal Psychology* 83, no. 3 (1974): 253–60.

Karuna Datta, Manjari Tripathi, Mansi Verma, Deepika Masiwal, and Hruda Nanda Mallick, "Yoga Nidra Practice Shows Improvement in Sleep in Patients with Chronic Insomnia: A Randomized Controlled Trial," *National Medical Journal of India* 34, no. 3 (2021): 143–150.

Maher Souabni, Mehdi J. Souabni, Omar Hammouda, Mohamed Romdhani, Khaled Trabelsi, Achraf Ammar, and Tarak Driss, "Benefits and Risks of Napping in Older Adults: A Systematic Review," *Frontiers in Aging Neuroscience* 14 (2022): 1000707.

American College of Sports Medicine, *ACSM's Guidelines for Exercise Testing and Prescription,* 10th Edition (2019): Updates to Tables 4.4 and 4.5.

Kevin D. Hall, Gary Sacks, Dalia Chandramohan, Carson D. Chow, Youfa Wang, Steven N. Gortmaker, and Boyd A. Swinburn, "Energy Balance and Its Components: Implications for Body Weight Regulation," *American Journal of Clinical Nutrition* 95, no. 4 (2012): 989–994.

Camila L. P. Oliveira, Normand G. Boulé, Arya M. Sharma, Sarah Elliott, Mario Siervo, Sunita Ghosh, Aloys Berg, and Carla M. Prado, "Examining the Effects of a High-Protein Total Diet Replacement on Energy Metabolism, Metabolic Blood Markers, and Appetite Sensations in Healthy Adults: Protocol for Two Complementary, Randomized, Controlled, Crossover Trials," *Trials* 20, no. 1 (2024): 787.

Cara B. Ebbeling, Henry A. Feldman, Gloria L. Klein, Julia M. W. Wong, Lisa Bielak, Sarah K. Steltz, Patricia K. Luoto, William W. Wong, and David S. Ludwig, "Effects of a Low Carbohydrate Diet on Energy Expenditure during Weight Loss Maintenance: Randomized Trial," *British Medical Journal* 363 (2018): k4583.

Nisa M. Maruthur, Scott J. Pilla, Karen White, Beiwen Wu, May Thu Thu Maw, Daisy Duan, Ruth-Alma Turkson-Ocran, Di Zhao, Jeanne Charleston, Courtney M. Peterson, Ryan J. Dougherty, Jennifer A. Schrack, Lawrence J. Appel, Eliseo Guallar, and Jeanne M. Clark, "Effect of Isocaloric, Time-Restricted Eating on

Body Weight in Adults With Obesity: A Randomized Controlled Trial," *Annals of Internal Medicine* 177, no. 5 (2024): 549–558.

Mai Severinsen, Charlotte Krogh, and Bente Klarlund Pedersen, "Muscle-Organ Crosstalk: The Emerging Roles of Myokines," *Endocrine Reviews* 41, no. 4 (2020): 594–609.

Beate E. M. Zunner, Nadine B. Wachsmuth, Max L. Eckstein, Lukas Scherl, Janis R Schierbauer, Sandra Haupt, Christian Stumpf, Laura Reusch, and Othmar Moser, "Myokines and Resistance Training: A Narrative Review," *International Journal of Molecular Sciences* 23, no. 7 (2022): 3501.

P. B. Gastin, "Energy System Interaction and Relative Contribution During Maximal Exercise," *Sports Medicine* (Auckland, N.Z.) 31, no. 10 (2001): 725–41.

Marco Romagnoli, Rafael Alis, Fabian Sanchis-Gomar, Giuseppe Lippi, and Alessandro Arduini, "An Eighteen-Minute Submaximal Exercise Test to Assess Cardiac Fitness in Response to Aerobic Training," *Journal of Strength and Conditioning Research* 32, no. 10 (2014): 2846–2852.

T-M Asikainen, S. Miilunpalo, P. Oja, M. Rinne, M. Pasanen, and I. Vuori, "Walking Trials in Postmenopausal Women: Effect of One vs Two Daily Bouts on Aerobic Fitness," *Scandinavian Journal of Medicine & Science in Sports* 12, no. 2 (2002): 99–105.

Barbara Strasser and Martin Burtscher, "Survival of the Fittest: VO2max, a Key Predictor of Longevity?" *Frontiers in Bioscience* 23, no. 8 (2018): 1505–1516.

Julio Morales and K. Fallon, "Relationship Between Training Load and Intensity and Next Day Resting Heart Rate in Running," *Medicine and Science in Sports and Exercise* 51, no. 6S (2019): Abstract 1047.

CHAPTER 8

Roy Chan, "Supporting Student Success Through Time and Technology," National Center on Time & Learning, U.S. Department of Education, 2012.

Frank Kellenberg, Joel T. Schmidt, and Christian Werner, "The Adult Learner: Self-Determined, Self-Regulated, and Reflective," *Signum Temporis* 9, no. 1 (2017): 23–29.

Matthew K. Nock, Michelle M. Wedig, Elizabeth B. Holmberg, and Jill M. Hooley, "The Emotion Reactivity Scale: Development, Evaluation, and Relation to Self-Injurious Thoughts and Behaviors," *Behavior Therapy* 39, no. 2 (2008): 107–116.

m. c. schraefel, George Catalin Muresan, and Eric Hekler, "Experiment in a Box (XB): An Interactive Technology Framework for Sustainable Health Practices," *Frontiers in Computer Science* 3 (2021).

m. c. schraefel and Eric Hekler, "Tuning: An Approach for Supporting Healthful Adaptation," *Interactions* 27, no. 2 (2020): 48–53.

PERSONAL HEALTH EXPERIMENTS

Harvard Emotional Reactivity Scale

Perceived Stress Scale

For each question choose from the following alternatives:

0 - never   1 - almost never   2 - sometimes   3 - fairly often   4 - very often

_____ 1. In the last month, how often have you been upset because of something that happened unexpectedly?

_____ 2. In the last month, how often have you felt that you were unable to control the important things in your life?

_____ 3. In the last month, how often have you felt nervous and stressed?

_____ 4. In the last month, how often have you felt confident about your ability to handle your personal problems?

_____ 5. In the last month, how often have you felt that things were going your way?

_____ 6. In the last month, how often have you found that you could not cope with all of the things that you had to do?

_____ 7. In the last month, how often have you been able to control irritations in your life?

_____ 8. In the last month, how often have you felt that you were on top of things?

_____ 9. In the last month, how often have you been angered because of things that happened that were outside of your control?

_____ 10. In the last month, how often have you felt difficulties were piling up so high that you could not overcome them?

Figuring Your PSS Score

You can determine your PSS score by following these directions:

- First, reverse your scores for questions 4, 5, 7, and 8. On these four questions, change the scores like this:
  0 = 4, 1 = 3, 2 = 2, 3 = 1, 4 = 0.

- Now add up your scores for each item to get a total: _____.

- Individual scores on the PSS can range from 0 to 40, with higher scores indicating higher perceived stress.

  - Scores ranging from 0–13 would be considered low stress.

  - Scores ranging from 14–26 would be considered moderate stress.

  - Scores ranging from 27–40 would be considered high stress.

Food Tracking Apps

MyFitnessPal
- Best for: General users and athletes
- Features:
  - Huge food database (millions of foods, barcode scanning)
  - Custom macronutrient goals and meal tracking
  - Syncs with fitness apps (Apple Health, FitBit, Garmin)
- Pros: Free version available, easy to use
- Cons: Some advanced features require premium subscription

Cronometer
- Best for: Precision tracking and micronutrients
- Features:
  - Highly accurate food database (lab-verified)
  - Tracks vitamins, minerals, and macronutrients
  - Great for ketogenic and low-carb diets
- Pros: More accurate than MyFitnessPal
- Cons: Smaller database than competitors

Carbon Diet—my personal favorite
- Best for: Athletes and bodybuilders
- Features:
  - Designed by Layne Norton, PhD
  - Dynamic macro adjustments based on progress
  - Custom goal setting: muscle gain, fat loss, or maintenance
- Pros: Science-backed macro coaching
- Cons: Subscription required, no free version

Inside Tracker
- Best for: Elite athletes, biohackers, and longevity-focused individuals
- Features:
  - Blood biomarker analysis: Measures glucose, cholesterol, inflammation, hormone levels, vitamins, and more
  - DNA-based insights: Identifies genetic predispositions for metabolism, recovery, and performance
  - Personalized nutrition and supplement recommendations: Based on blood work and lifestyle data
  - Integrates with fitness and nutrition apps: Syncs with Apple Health, Garmin, FitBit, and MyFitnessPal
- Pros: AI-driven health coaching: Provides custom strategies for sleep, stress, recovery, and training
- Cons:
  - No built-in calorie and macro tracking (must integrate with other apps)
  - Expensive—biomarker testing ranges from $100 to $600 per test
  - Not necessary for casual users—better suited for high-performance athletes

INDEX

digest, in parasympathetic nervous system (PSNS), 90
discipline, 270–273
distal tools, 76–79
doomscrolling, 216
Dual Energy X-ray Absorptiometry (DEXA) scans
    about, 231–232
    for Body Composition experiment, 366–367
Dumas, Alexander, 20
dumbbells, 234–235
Durham, Zee, 123

E

earplugs, 217
eating
    MTTR and, 255
    for muscle mass and body composition, 236–237
    sleep and, 213–214
Edison, Thomas, 220
education, process of change and, 279
electroencephalography (EEG), 205
emotional layer, in Triune Brain model, 94–101
emotional processing, during REM and NREM sleep, 201
emotional scales, 116
emotional thinking, 98–99
emotional tools, for stress, 110
emotional valence, 96
Emotional Well-Being experiment, 312–317

end range isometrics, 166
energy, 238–243
Engineers, 266–269
enrichment, sleep and, 221–222
ethics, emotions and, 98–99
executive function, 102–104
exercise, sleep and, 218–219
experience, researching your own, 291–294
"Experiment in a Box (XB): An Interactive Technology Framework for Sustainable Health Practices" (schrafel), 286–287
experimental mindset, developing, 285
exteroception, 30
extraversion, as a personality domain, 9–10

F

feeding window, 370
feeling states, effects of early experiences on, 99–100
feelings
    costs of, 100–101
    history of, 95–97
Feldenkrais Method, 172
Few, Stephen, *Information Dashboard Design*, 59
fiber intake, as a tool for Body Composition experiment, 369–370
fight, in sympathetic nervous system (SNS), 90
first responder work, 203–204

V

Vehicle Dependability Study (VDS), 73
Vesalius, Andreas, 188
vestibular system, 132
video games, 279–280
Virginia High Performance, 77
visceral fat, 224
visual system, 132
volume oxygen maximum (VO2) max
    about, 243
    for Aerobic Health experiment, 378

W

walking, as a tool for Aerobic Health experiment, 383
Wall Push, as a tool for Isometrics experiment, 329–330
Warrior Fitness Program, 10–11
wearables
    about, 47, 58
    MIND and, 93–94
    sleep and, 199–200, 205, 206
    zooming in/out and, 263
Wilson, Rob, personal story of, 17–21
wind-down routine, 202
women
    fiber intake for, 369
    muscle mass and, 229–230
    2-kilometer walk test for, 380
working memory, 103

Y

yoga, 179, 180–182
Yoga Nidra, 220

Z

Zinkowski, Cheryl, 365
Zinn, Jon Kabat, 121
Zone 2 training, 245–246
zooming in/out, 263–266

ABOUT THE AUTHOR

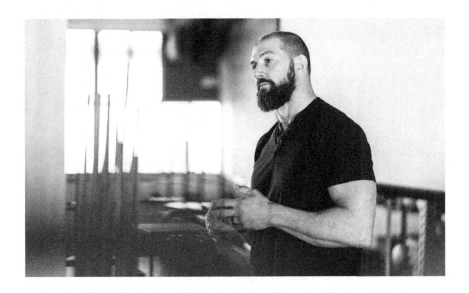

Rob Wilson is a human performance specialist with over twenty years of manual therapy, coaching, and education experience. His work spans a variety of avenues in the fields of health and human performance. This includes multiple trademarks, the creation of global seminars and curriculums, and the research, development, and implementation of best practices in human performance.

Over the past three years, Rob has created and led his Check Engine Light curriculum, working with more than 600 active duty and veteran special operators. He also works with professional athletes, corporate executives, and first responders, helping them enhance performance longevity, resilience, and recovery. Rob has been a pioneer in the research and development of breath control practices for health and high-level performance. He has contributed ideas and presented to the best of the best, including the UFC Performance Institute, ALTIS, and the U.S. and Allied Special Forces.

Rob is an avid martial artist and surfer as well as a devoted husband and father. When he's not nose-deep in research, you can find him on the mat or with his wife and their many animals.

Victory Belt Publishing
3145 W Torino Ave.
US-NV, 89118
US
https://www.victorybelt.com
859-663-8017

The authorized representative in the EU for product safety and compliance is

YoBo Graphics Ltd
Boryana Vasileva Yordanova
26 Bulair Str.
ECZ, 4000
BG
yobo@victorybelt.com

ISBN: 9781628605440
Release ID: 151969226

Made in the USA
Las Vegas, NV
04 July 2025

24447975R00246